MW00623615

The Thermo Diet: How To Eat

Christopher Walker is the co-founder and CEO of UMZU. He is the first person to graduate from Duke University's neuroscience program in just 3 years, while studying a range of topics from endocrinology, to neuroeconomics, learning & memory, neurobiology, physics, and AI. Christopher's obsession with human nature and biology helped him heal all of the symptoms of his brain tumor naturally, without drugs or surgery. Disgusted with his negative experiences with the medical establishment, Christopher has spent the past decade creating natural health solutions, products, and educational resources, teaching millions of men and women around the world how to use nutrition, strategic supplementation, and physical training to heal their nagging health issues naturally. His guiding philosophy is that your body is a self-healing organism, you just need to allow it to help itself.

"Thermo is honestly a cheat code." - *Tyler Stephens, Florida*

"I love the Thermo Diet! I hate to even call it a diet! I started 6 weeks ago and I'm already down 9 pounds. Amazing to me especially since I have Hashimoto's and losing weight for me is near to impossible." - *Cassia Sturgeon, Arizona*

"I wanted to say a big thank you to Christopher Walker and his team. I'm not 100% sure what my weight was when I started (between 195 and 200), but I hit 180 this week, which is a weight I've not seen in 11 or 12 years. I've also lost 4 inches off my waist. And, I struggled with acid reflux for years and years, and I've been taking a prescription drug for that every other day for about a year. Since starting Thermo, acid reflux has disappeared, and I don't remember the last time I took a pharmaceutical." - *Chris Huddleston, West Virginia*

"I lost 50 pounds and gained muscle while following the philosophies in The Thermo Diet. I was surprised at how steady fat loss was during the whole process because usually, I plateau at some point. Making sure my hormones were balanced and removing all micronutrient deficiencies definitely played a role in keeping my metabolism high."- *Zach Siegel, Colorado*

"The biggest results for me have been less bloating and an overall healthier relationship with food! I used to really limit my sugar and carb intake, rarely even eating fruit - so this "diet" has been liberating! I joined this for health, not necessarily to lose weight so I've just been maintaining, but it has helped me lose inches already from just bloat. Love it!" - *Emily Saviano, California*

"I've dealt with stomach issues and indigestion problems for years and Thermo has completely changed my life. Love the UMZU products, love this lifestyle, love Christopher Walker." - *Hayley Jacques, California*

"Honestly I've felt amazing in the morning again when I break the fast with organic fruit and coffee. The first few days were hard but now I can't wait to get up and slice some organic pears, apples, oranges, and berries!" - *Candace Bogue*

"I used to believe that low carb was necessary to have steady energy throughout the day. But since going Thermo and increasing my carbs dramatically, specifically from white rice, potatoes, and fruit I have a lot better energy. It really shines in the gym where I could literally feel the difference. My strength improved and my muscles are a lot fuller. After a couple weeks of eating Thermo I have incredible sustained energy with no spikes or drops." - *Matt Hayes, Michigan*

"I feel great on Thermo! More energy and less cravings." - *Athena Mayorga Blude, Connecticut*

"My sex drive is absolutely through the roof. I can easily pack on muscle at the gym; it seems like every other week I can hit new PRs. And my energy levels are super high - being a 34 year old father of 2, working 2 jobs, coaching both my kids year round, I actually find it super easy to have enough energy to do this." - *Jake Miner, Wisconsin*

"Thermo is basically my dream diet. I remember feeling so bloated all the time, I had no energy, I was always exhausted, and I just couldn't understand why I was having all those feelings because I was working out 4-5 times per week, and I had just run my second marathon. Even after all that training I had only ever lost like 3-5 pounds... I was eating what I thought at the time was very "healthy" but I couldn't ever drop the weight. So my husband told me about Chris and the Thermo Lifestyle, and I thought "well, what's the worst that could possibly happen?"" - *Rachel Siebold, California*

"Thermo seems like a better all around balanced diet. I've done keto and bulletproof diets in the past. They did work to some degree but also had drawbacks. I was strict keto for a year and never got down low enough body fat to have clear abs. First time in my life now I have a killer six pack and that's with getting 200g+ carbs a day with Thermo." - *Josh Webb, Michigan*

"My energy is back. I actually feel motivated to work out every day now! That hasn't happened to me in over 2 years." - *Jonathan Schrager, Florida*

"I tried the ketogenic diet and it messed up my metabolic rate, constantly tired, no energy, low libido and moodiness. When I went Thermo and started incorporating strategic carbs from fruit, rice, and potatoes everything improved. I can't explain how much more energy I have throughout the day." - *Alex Fidurski, Ireland*

"Following the guidelines that I have discovered through the Thermo Diet, I experienced increased energy, and overall my health has dramatically increased. I utilized these principles to lose fat while preparing for my competition and simultaneously taking care of my health. If it wasn't for Thermo I would be in shambles right now from contest dieting." - *Tim Berlow, Arizona*

"Eating for hormones has been the best choice I have made, period. Thanks to all you Thermo Warriors. Beneath the body has legitimately been a mind transformation, one that occurs with natural hormonal balances. Friends and family have noticed and honestly, good real food is the way to go!" - *Adam Little, Kuwait*

"My hair was going south fast... and it wasn't just for the winter. I was only in my mid-20's. I was confused because I thought hair loss was only for older guys. At the time, I was on a vegan diet, with high soy consumption, and for a couple years before that I'd been on the Keto Diet. What I didn't realize was that those diets were completely destroying my health.

My hair was falling out by the handful! When I discovered the Thermo Diet way of eating I finally stopped losing my hair... and not only that, but I regrew ALL of my hair back, thicker than ever.

Now that I'm doing Thermo, it's growing like crazy, I have to cut it every 2-3 weeks. Follow these tips that I used and you'll be loving life again when your hair starts growing back. Lemme tell you, it's the best feeling ever." - *Aron Georgia-Keys, Australia*

The Simple Scientific Way To Eat To Heal Your Hormones, Lose Fat Easily, & Increase Your Metabolism Fast

THERMODIET™

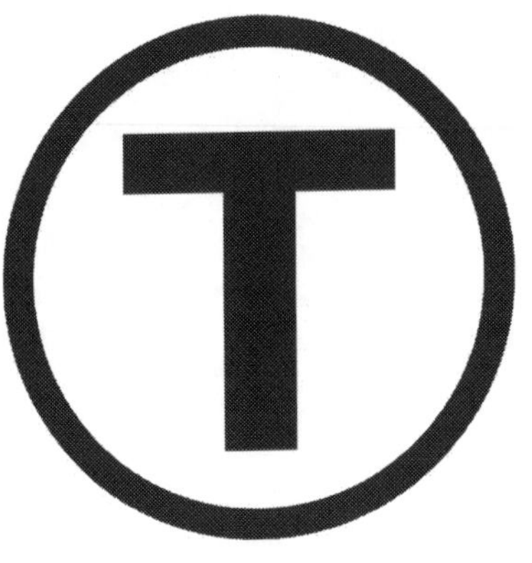

Christopher Walker

The Thermo Diet: How To Eat

Research Assistant: Jayton Miller

Graphics & Design: Zach Siegel & Brenton Leasure

ISBN 978-1-7370414-0-5 Hardcover

978-1-7370414-1-2 Paperback

978-1-7370414-3-6 Audiobook

978-1-7370414-2-9 Ebook

This book is dedicated to you, the curious reader. May you be inspired to use the knowledge and stories herein to become a better version of yourself.

Acknowledgements

I am grateful to a handful of great scientific and philosophical thinkers, clearly ahead of their time, who have inspired me over the years with their writing. Writing can be a thankless task, but while I read your words silently, they resounded loudly inside my mind. Thanks to many of you for giving me information that served as clues to help me heal myself 10 years ago. Now I want to pay it forward by bringing my own book to the world, to hopefully propagate the truth further out of obscurity into the light of Understanding inside the minds of many more people who need it.

Dr. William J. Walsh, PhD., Dr. Raymond Peat PhD., Sir Francis Bacon, Dr. Broda Barnes M.D., Isaac Newton, Dr. Robert Lanza M.D., Erich Neumann, Jeffrey M. Schwartz, M.D., Eric Hoffer, Baltasar Gracian, Ralph Waldo Emerson, Robert Greene, Gustave Le Bon M.D., Rick Strassman M.D., Jeff S. Volek PhD. & William J. Kramer PhD., Antonio Damasio M.D. PhD. and to my Duke University professors who helped reignite a love of learning & curiosity in me and countless other students Ingrid Byerly PhD., Scott Huettel PhD., Henry Yin PhD., Lawrence E. Evans PhD., J. Edward Ladenburger M.S., and Craig Roberts PhD.

And an especially big thank you to my family. To my uncle Dr. Richard Olson M.D. for always supporting my curiosity to learn about the human body. To my Father and Mother for instilling a tenacious work ethic in me through your own example, allowing me to be myself, and follow my internal compass. And my brother Robert and sister Katherine, for continually inspiring me with your own internal drive & integrity.

And to my business partners and ***UMZU*** team, for trusting my vision and your drive to wake up every day to create the better future we all see so clearly.

"Books ought to have no patrons but Truth and Reason." *- Sir Francis Bacon*

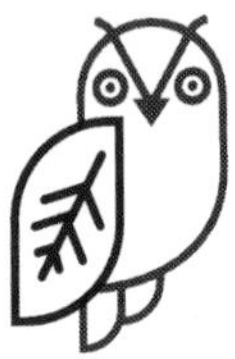

Contents

Preface

When I was 19 I was diagnosed with a brain tumor.

I had begun my freshman year pre-med at Duke University to get my degree in neuroscience, but I was having some seriously strange issues. I rapidly lost so much weight that I looked like a skeleton, yet I had no appetite. I was having trouble getting out of bed in the morning, let alone focusing in class, my brain completely numb, like I was floating in a constant haze, severely depressed for no discernable reason whatsoever.

My joints were also aching so badly that I started taking an over-the-counter NSAID daily called Aleve to reduce the pain, a terrible decision that landed me in the Duke Hospital ICU for a week after the student health center discovered that I had developed severe acute internal bleeding from 3 gaping ulcers in my duodenum, losing enough blood through my stool to nearly go into hemorrhagic shock.

Things got so hopeless that I had to take a medical leave of absence for my entire sophomore year.

During that year, my doctors gave me antidepressants and put me into a behavioral therapy program at Mary Washington Hospital in northern Virginia. I felt like I was going insane because I truly had no clue what was going on in my head, but for the previous couple years I'd been experiencing crippling symptoms and could barely function in my daily life.

It wasn't until more than 6 months of therapy and drug treatments that I finally went into the doctor's office and begged him for a blood test.

No tests had been run prior to that day, but I knew something was horribly wrong with my body.

My "tip-off" was the fact that I hadn't had a sex drive in nearly 2 years. Zip. Nada. Zilch.

No libido whatsoever.

As a 17-19 year old guy... that's not normal.

The doctor relented, and finally (albeit reluctantly) gave me the blood test I asked for.
One glance at the results, and his eyes were as big as dinner plates.

"I'm going to have to send you to a specialist," he said.

I was sent to a hematologist/oncologist in Potomac, Virginia, where the specialist ran a comprehensive blood and hormone panel.

Within 30 seconds of looking at the results, he turned to me and said, *"I think you have a brain tumor. I need to order an MRI."*

The MRI confirmed it, a tumor in my pituitary, sitting at the base of my brain, blocking critical hormone production and signaling to the body.

I remember thinking, *"What a relief! I'm not insane!"*

A light switch turned on in my mind when I saw that MRI result... There is a biological basis for my entire experience in life: my behavior, all of my health issues, my worldview. It's ALL rooted in my biology and can be influenced by biological function, and dysfunction.

My battle with the medical establishment had begun.
My entire experience leading up to the tumor discovery and diagnosis was infuriating! Instead of giving me a simple blood test, my doctor was quick to prescribe me pharmaceuticals and check me into a hospital therapy program for 6 months!

How backwards is that? I had to get the blood test by eventually demanding it myself. Only then, with real biological data, did the doctor see that this was a much more serious issue than he thought, and I needed real help.

After the diagnosis, I was given two options. First, was surgery. Due to the positioning of the tumor behind the optic nerve, and the risk associated with a surgical blunder (ie. blindness), I did not want to surgically remove the tumor unless it was an absolute necessity for survival.

I opted for his second option, to monitor its growth every 6 months with MRIs, and to use hormone replacement therapies and antidepressants for the rest of my life, and to see a psychiatrist monthly to renew my prescriptions.

After just a few weeks on the drug cocktail, I was feeling just as terrible as before. To my doctors' dismay (and probably my parents' as well at the time) I refused to continue taking the pharmaceuticals, and threw them in the trash. As I walked out of my psychiatrist's office after telling her I wasn't going to continue my prescriptions, I distinctly remember her saying, *"you're making a huge mistake."*

It didn't make any sense to me that I would have to use these drugs for the rest of my life. Why didn't anybody even think about natural ways to help my body heal itself? The body is a self-healing organism when it has the resources it needs to do so. This was never even considered as an option by any of the doctors I talked to.

I'd realized that nobody cared about my health as much as I did - a truth I think everyone should accept for themselves.

I returned to Duke in the fall for my junior year, with a tenacious obsession to finish my neuroscience degree in 3 years instead of 4 (I became the first person to ever complete the program that quickly) and to use all of the world-class resources at my disposal for that final 2 years to solve my health problems naturally.

And guess what...

I did.

Within 18 months I'd completely, naturally, fixed all of the hormonal issues the tumor had been causing for years. I even brought my testosterone levels up from 11 ng/dL to 1192 ng/dL with just food, supplements, and specific exercise habits - a feat all conventional medical "wisdom" would deem impossible.

The tumor was still in my brain, the same size, but I was able to completely override its negative effects through just smart nutrition and lifestyle optimization.
I remember knowing I could do this, when I learned about the concept of feedback-loops in the human endocrine system. These self-reinforcing hormone signaling loops can amplify your results when positive input is continually fed into them, making hormone optimization easier and easier, which in my case, eventually overpowered the signaling block the tumor was causing in my pituitary.

Hormones are the most powerful chemical compounds inside

our bodies, and when optimized can rapidly turn your health around and bring you into a state of vibrant energy and balance, a state I now refer to as *Thermo*.

My original plan to be a neurosurgeon never came to fruition - I was too disgusted with the medical system to allow myself to participate in it. The institutional dogma is too deeply entrenched, with most modern medical practices completely centered around pharmaceutical distribution. My fascination with, and love of, the human body grew to such a profound level of respect that I could not willingly indenture myself to a system that is set up only to medicate patients, not to actually help them solve the root causes of their health problems safely and naturally, which empowers the patient to prevent further issues in the future. I graduated with my degree in 2011 and left academia forever.

I started writing about my story online back in 2012 and never really intended for my blogging to be much more than an outlet for me to share my knowledge with people, and help them avoid a similar fate.

However, destiny has had other plans.

Apparently my experience was not unique. Millions of men, women, & kids around the world have had similar let-down experiences with the medical system, and are actively searching for help online. Many of them found my writing, and over the subsequent years I've owned health websites that get millions of searching visitors every month, and my health videos and podcasts on social media have averaged over 100 million views/ listens per year for years now.

I never thought this would snowball into such a cool, important thing! But not everybody's heard the good word yet, so I've got a lot of work still left to do.

In 2015 I decided to start my company UMZU, to formulate and make the highest quality natural supplements possible, all backed with scientific research & ingredients with human clinical trials, and dosed correctly for people to use to help give their body the nutrients - the raw materials - it needs in order to start its self-healing process.

I'm proud to say that we've helped hundreds of thousands of customers so far, allowing for many of them to get off their dangerous pharmaceuticals by using natural, well-formulated supplements. We serve people all over the world, shipping our products out from our Boulder Colorado facilities.

And this is just the beginning. With my amazing team and business partners, I plan to build UMZU into the #1 natural products company in the world.

This book you're holding in your hands is vital for you to read and understand.

Within these pages lie the simple secrets to a more perfect state of human health. No 'biohacks,' tricks, or shortcuts. Just a foundationally true examination of how our bodies work paired with nutrition recommendations to help your body function properly.

It's not boring either. I'm a big fan of learning the historical basis of our current reality, especially when it comes to suppressed, or hidden, history. It's like pulling the thread out of an endless sweater. I will walk you through some of the truly backwards, fucked up, stories that spawned our modern ideas of nutrition and health... how things came to be the way they are now.

Follow the steps, enjoy the stories, absorb the information, and make it a way of life. Your health will improve rapidly, and with surprisingly little effort, once you accept the simple truths you're about to read.

I am obsessed with understanding the truth and my hope is that this will be self-evident as you read this book. *There are no sacred cows when it comes to discerning fact from fiction, especially when it comes to something as important as your health.*

We all need to be healthy in order to perform our best. The current conventional health paradigm isn't cutting it for anybody. Don't think you're unique in your struggles; we're all in this boat together. And it's time to start rowing ourselves.

The nutrition recommendations you're about to learn are

currently being used by high-performers and Average Janes & Joe's alike. By simply opening this book, you're ahead of the curve. Start absorbing and applying this information and you'll instantly be light years ahead.

If you're ready to start getting real, lasting results, you've found the right book.

Cheers to your health Thermo Warrior,

Christopher Walker
UMZU.com

Silent majority
Raised by the system
Now it's time to rise against...

- Pennywise "Fuck Authority"

The healers have become the harmers
They're just pharmaceutical farmers
What we used to call dealers
We now call doctors.

- NOFX, "Oxy Moronic"

Introduction To Thermo

Your current state of health directly influences your experience in the world. Think about it: if you're overweight right now, even if you only have about 15-20lbs to lose, your experience of the world is much different from the experience you'd be living if you didn't have that extra body fat. This is not meant to be mean, so much as to allow you an opportunity to consider something.

There are infinite different versions of yourself. Every present moment, you're choosing to step into one of these versions. These choices could be a progression, or a digression. But ultimately, the direction you move in always comes down to your choices.

Patterns develop, and these patterns become your habits. If you're currently 200lbs, for example, and you have about 20lbs to lose before you feel lean, fit, and healthy - I can assure you, the habit patterns that the 180lb version of yourself has are different from your current 200lb self's habit patterns.

Usually they're not that drastically different, but they do require a new direction of action in certain high leverage areas of your daily choices. The beautiful thing is this: you can choose, at any moment, to step into the habit patterns of your 180lb self. When you make that choice, and reinforce it daily, in time you will eventually become that 180lb version of yourself. All this requires is a visualization, a path to follow to reach that outcome.

In this book, I provide you with this clear path. Armed with clarity and understanding, execution will become natural. It will no longer be forced.

Have you ever felt like every diet or nutrition plan you've tried has been an uphill battle?

Maybe in the first week or two, fresh with motivation to start anew, you do well on your plan, but by the third week you've already "fallen off the wagon?" Don't worry this is all too common. Basically everyone does it. But why?

The chief reason for this is the fact that the action is not coupled with clarity or understanding.

"Action" typically associated with an individual following a fad diet or a crash diet always comes from a place of desperation – and often even fear or boredom – albeit usually backed by a good intention. And therein lies the root of the failure: the individual's mind is not ready for the journey. It has not stepped into the requirements that are needed to become that better version. Their mind *agrees* with the idea, but does not truly *understand* the requirements for it.

True understanding is always coupled with action.

The first thing I want you to understand as you embark on this Thermo Diet journey above all else is that your mental game matters.

You need to level up your mental game so that you can succeed on this program "without even trying" - which really means, in a thoroughly enjoyable way. It won't feel like "dieting" because it isn't; it's lifestyle adjustment and mental engineering.

This is not an uphill battle, it's going to be like floating downstream in a relaxing river. But you have to get your mind right first.

Second, I want you to understand and accept that improving your internal environment, both physiological and psychological, will manifest in outward improvements in your physique and energy throughout the day.

As you become healthier on a cellular level, the amount of energy your body produces is going to make you feel incredible. You will not only become more successful in your career and relationships because of this, but your physique is also going to improve since you'll be working with your body to flow in the direction it wants. Your body wants to be lean, fit, energetic, and strong. You just need to allow it to do so.

As you improve your biology and psychology, your reality is going to improve to reflect this progress.

It's a universal law; it's simple; and it works.

What Is Thermo?

Thermo is your body's natural state of vibrant health.

One of the fundamental truths of biology is the fact that your body is always working to restore homeostasis. This homeostasis, on the level of the human organism, is a state of perfect health: a fast metabolism, a lean body, strong muscle tissue, and fully functioning sexual organs.

To my awareness, nobody has ever coined a term for this state of health in humans, so I am taking the liberty of doing that right now, with the word Thermo. Any time I refer to it throughout this book, you'll know what I am referencing. The Thermo Diet is a way of eating and living that supports bringing your body back into the Thermo State.

The purpose of this program is to show you the path to your Thermo State - a path that is surprisingly simple, when you get out of your own way.

This book asks and answers the following questions:

1.) What is The Thermo Diet?

The Thermo Diet is a way of nourishing your body to help it slip back into the downstream flow of restoring itself to the Thermo State: a lean, fit, strong physique, with full sexual health, clarity of mind, and boundless energy.

When most people picture themselves with all of these traits, it hearkens back to the times of their youth - typically their teenage years - long before the negative effects of poor nutrition, stress, environmental toxins, and other manners of adult "life" began to manifest. These are usually the traits that we most long for as we age. We long to have them restored. We long for them, precisely because we've tasted their sweet nectar, and the freedom inherent in them, before.

However, sadly most of us don't realize that we can have these traits once again. That our bodies naturally want to restore us to this state once again. This book is going to teach you exactly what to do to restore this level of vibrant health back into your life. When you nourish your body to support its natural biochemistry, and eliminate key "blockers" from your life that are holding your body back, keeping it sick, you will quickly restore yourself to Thermo.

2.) *Is The Thermo Diet For Anybody?*

Yes, this way of eating is suited for men, women, and children. It's scientifically sound, non-restrictive, and will not lead to deficiencies, cravings, or neuroticism - as most other diets will. In fact, The Thermo Diet is designed to literally be the opposite of these things. Its purpose is to nourish your body from the cellular level up through the organism level so thoroughly that deficiencies - either physiological (ie. micronutrient and macronutrient) or psychological (perceived restriction always leads to binge/purge cycles) - will become a thing of the past.

3.) Why Is Thermo Essential?

You're going to discover why Thermo is so important for getting the body and health that looks as good on the inside as it does on the outside. You're going to discover that many of those traits I mentioned earlier (a lean, fit, strong physique, with full sexual health, clarity of mind, and boundless energy) that most of us struggle to restore, and therefore give up on, are actually innate emergent properties of your body's natural state. You desire these traits for a reason! Your body and mind do not want to be sick, fat, impotent, and depressed. I hope that's not a shocking thing to realize.

4.) How does Thermo work, and how can you get it to work for you?

You're going to be introduced to the bioenergetics model of the natural capacity for energy production on the cellular level that every person is born with. This innate process generates 100% of the energy used in your body every single second of every day. Ultimately, the health of this system is paramount to your health in general. It dictates the way your body looks, the way you feel, how clearly you think, and therefore how you move through, and experience, the world.

Thermo is a natural emergent property of human bioenergetics - it isn't something you do, it's something you already have. Like I mentioned before, it's a natural state that most of us have been actively fighting against since our teenage years through "blockers" such as stress, poor nutrition, and exposure to environmental toxins. Your body has its own "self-clearing" functions, capable of guiding you back to the Thermo State, regardless of what state or circumstances your body may be in currently. While this Thermo State is highly evident in youth, all but a fortunate few have "blocked" this vibrant health from continuing into adulthood.

As you start to deepen your understanding of human bioenergetics, you're going to reconnect with your body's natural self-clearing function. As a result, you'll find that you start having a). Natural, almost effortless body fat loss b). Clear, direct thinking (no more brain fog) c). An insatiable sexual appetite once again d). Incredible energy throughout the day and in the gym e). Stronger muscle tissue with visibly defined muscular structure. Some other "side effects" may include low stress, no more anxiety or depression, the ability to sleep restfully through the night, and the disappearance of food cravings.

5.) Why do we need Thermo now more than ever?

We're living in a pivotal point in history. The dissemination of information has never been so widespread or so fast. This has enabled some absolutely incredible advancements in human understanding and research. It's also opened the door for misinformation to spread like a virus.

If ignorance was a disease, it's never been easier to "catch." The very fact that you're going through this book right now points to the reality that you've likely seen many many other books, articles, and videos on nutrition plans and other diets.

But the reason you're reading this one, at this very moment, is likely because *those programs didn't work for you.* They didn't serve you. Sure, maybe some aspects of them were good, but other aspects were bad. And ultimately, in the end, it was all unsustainable, causing you to look elsewhere for help. Right now, you can rest assured that you've found what you need. The information you're about to absorb will give you the "aha" moment you've been craving. The missing piece to the puzzle.

Not only that, but disease is on the rise like never before. It seems like nearly everyone contracts some form of cancer, autoimmune disease, or metabolic syndrome at one point or another these days. This should be a massive warning sign! Alarm bells are ringing.

The current way we're eating and living, the toxins and drugs we're exposing ourselves to, are prematurely killing us. And if the original disease doesn't kill us quickly, the side effects from all the pharmaceutical "therapies" we are prescribed will become more than just nagging annoyances, typically requiring even further medication to alleviate their effects, dragging us slowly-but-surely, face down in the mud behind the pale horse.

I obviously don't want this for anyone. I'm here with this book to help break you free from the vicious cycle you're in. To empower you to think for yourself, and to take back control over your health once again.

"The miracle of self-healing occurs when the inner patient yields to the inner physician."
- Vernon Howard

One of the main things that we're proud of at our company UMZU, is that we have developed a health philosophy that's based on human biochemistry, and that is focused on following the right steps to allow for your body to heal itself from the inside out.

Very few companies will ever take the time to develop a system like this for their products, opting instead to just sell anything under the sun, regardless of if it actually helps the customer or not.

In fact, we do the opposite. We actually developed our natural healing philosophies years BEFORE creating our products, and we now build supplemental formulas around supporting our customers on their healing journey. This, we believe, is the proper - and most effective - way to serve the customer and build a great, long-lasting company and community.

You might be wondering, *"Well, I'm not sick. I'm not wounded. Why would I need to heal myself?"*

That's a good question, and a very common misunderstanding among the average person.

Because the truth is, **you *are* sick.** We are all deficient in key micronutrients, we're exposed to endocrine disrupting chemicals constantly - not to mention, we're adding unnecessary stimuli, foods, and stressors to our bodies that are getting in the way of our innate self-healing capacities - and our bodies are consequently operating below our real capacity to thrive.

Imagine... just some small tweaks in these areas and your body's ability to produce energy will multiply. Your metabolism will increase quickly, turning you into a fat-burning furnace of high-energy cells. Body fat will naturally, and rather quickly, burn as fuel, revealing your true physique.

Imagine... the mental clarity and focus increase when your brain is operating on all cylinders, not just because it's being fed it's preferred fuel source and has all the key vitamins and minerals it needs for neurotransmission, but also because the gut microbiome is supplying a direct line of feedback to it for hormone regulation and micronutrient replenishment.

When the body starts to enter the Thermo State, it's self-healing capacity is operating seamlessly. And as a welcome side-effect, you start to experience other benefits like body fat loss, physique transformation, and boundless energy throughout the day.

This is all achievable without restricting carbs, fats, or proteins, as many fad diets would have you do.

Carbohydrates, certain types of fats, and proteins are all necessary macronutrients for your body to truly thrive metabolically and hormonally, contrary to popular opinion. This is an irrefutable truth that I will delve deeper into later in this book so you can gain the necessary clarity around the topic of macronutrients.

One of the key failures of other diets you may have tried in the past is the fact that they put all their attention on things that don't matter. They put all their attention on restriction. They put all their attention on emotional arguments or conjecture. I prefer to use foundational truth.

Let's put all that garbage in the past, and move into an age of enlightenment around how the human body operates biochemically, and the true nutritional requirements it has in order to thrive and evolve upward to a state of higher functioning.

The ironic, but entirely logical, truth about this is that you cannot reach this evolved state of higher functioning without first restoring your body to its true Thermo State of being: *its natural state.* Only from this state of homeostatic nirvana will it be able to accelerate into a better place, not from the current state of sickness and deficiency that many of us find ourselves in.

The plan I am going to outline for you here is based on biochemistry. It's based on the science of YOUR body. This entire book is designed to outline 9 Laws Of Nutrition based on Thermo realities: how to eat and live in a way that will restore your body to the Thermo State quickly and painlessly.

Your body is not meant to carry excess fat tissue, especially not to the point of causing metabolic and hormonal damage to itself. And contrary to what most people would have you believe, the cause of the accumulation of this excess fat has far less to do with macronutrients, and much more to do with micronutrients and other small molecule exposure and bacterial imbalance.

This is good news. Armed with the knowledge and action plan in this book you will know how to eliminate all of the blockers from your life, and allow your body to seamlessly flow back into the Thermo State.

And the most exciting part about this is that, on a daily basis, you will be consuming meals that are satisfying, delicious, and make you feel as though you're not "dieting" at all... because if a "diet" is typically associated with restriction, then this is in fact not a diet at all. It's a lifestyle. And a thoroughly enjoyable one at that.

The Unifying Principle Of Bioenergetics

Bioenergetics is the idea that biology is based around and dependent on energy, and that by improving our energetic state, we can improve our biology - our health and well-being. We know this is true because matter, like your body, is simply condensed, or focused, energy via E=mc2.

You might find this to be a radical thought, but you don't "create" energy at all. Rather, energy is constantly flowing through systems, defining your physical body, from the cellular up to the organism levels.

All life starts and ends with energy. If you'll recall from your high school physics class, you'll remember the *First Law Of Thermodynamics: the Law Of Conservation Of Energy* that shows that energy cannot be created or destroyed in an isolated system.

This concept has been articulated throughout history, since ancient times. As long as humans have lived and had the capacity for critical thought, we've understood this truth in one form or another.

This energy is condensed into different forms of matter, some visible to the human eye and some invisible. Some of this matter is our body... our physical cells, tissues, organs. Our thoughts are forms of energy as well, albeit invisible. But they are unquestionably, just as real as our fingernails or knee caps. The fact that you're aware of reading this sentence right now is proof of that.

Energy is present across a vibrational spectrum. Nothing is at rest; everything is constantly vibrating, albeit at different wavelengths. Low energy states are characterized by low vibration frequency, high energy states are characterized by higher frequencies.

With higher vibration comes higher forms of order, higher levels of structure in a system.

This has been proven, for example, with the human brain itself, whereas through an evolutionary process the brain has become inexplicably intricate in structure, to the point of manifesting *The Hard Problem* of consciousness. The human brain has a multitude higher metabolic rate and energy flow than that of even other near-relative primates like chimpanzees.

The evolution to more complex forms of matter is due to this increase in energy moving through the system.

However, make no mistake about it, life is not an entitled progression... you can *devolve.*

And many people have. It is painfully obvious that some people operate on a higher frequency than others.

It is your choice to either continue this higher energy evolution or, on the other hand, to devolve into a lower energy state.

Your thoughts will influence this process, yes, however nutrition also plays an absolutely MASSIVE role in the energy flow through your body. Most people do not grasp the importance of feeding your body so it operates in a high energy state. The quality of food and the nutrients you consume are paramount to the cellular frequency you operate at.

Many people make daily nutritional choices that constantly input dissonance into the energetic frequency of their body, lowering the frequency into states of disease and fog, as opposed to health and clarity.

When you introduce, and reinforce, this dissonance via poor nutritional habits you are essentially forcing your cells into operating not as a cohesive unit with coherence throughout the organism, but as fractional units - as simpler life forms focused on survival.

Cancer is a perfect example of this, and probably the height of cellular dissonance and dysfunction in humans. Cancer cells act irrespective of the entire organism; in fact, they act in opposition to the organism, killing other cells, degrading tissue, causing more dysfunction throughout.

The concept of the "whole" is lost; therefore the whole dies prematurely.

When cells operate at low energy levels, with low frequency, your health as an organism degrades quickly. Typically this degradation is most evident in loss of hormonal function via an underperforming endocrine system. The cells are in survival mode, not focused on thriving and evolution, but rather on keeping the organism alive. Most people live in this survival mode due to choices and habits that they do not know are putting them there. However, other people intentionally make nutritional decisions, especially nowadays with certain fad diets that they think will lead to "quick fat loss" but are actually harming their cells' ability to thrive by shifting themselves into endocrine survival mode.

You thrive as an organism when your cells have high energy flow.

A by-product of this high energy state is a lean and healthy physique. Sadly, the average person has this backward: instead of focusing on building thriving systemic health via increasing energy flow, they chase "weight loss" by damaging their energy flow, through fad diets, macronutrient elimination, low nutrient diets, and stress induction.

Any fat loss through these methods is short lived. The *Law of Compensation* will always kick in, swinging the pendulum with brutal force and consequences for any shortcut seeking.

These concepts, undoubtedly may seem either difficult to grasp, or excessively grandiose for some people. Let me assure you, they are neither difficult nor grandiose; in fact, they're quite simple and foundational. These concepts I'm teaching you now are applicable on every level of life. They're universal. Unfortunately, we've been conditioned and educated by lazy minds on the topic of nutrition in the mainstream modern health industry: people limited to a scope of regurgitating information they've heard elsewhere, without much attention to foundational biology, and most definitely without the application of context and a search for the truth.

This has led to an entire population of confused, ill-informed, and diseased people.

Let's turn this ship around.

Fat loss, for example, is an easy place to begin since it is something most people are concerned with. Fat gain is a product of low energy flow from a slow metabolism.

Saying that obesity is an issue of low energy may seem counterintuitive at first, especially since most people consider fat gain to be a product of too much energy.

In reality the opposite is true - fat gain is a problem of lower cellular energy levels from a lower metabolism, despite adequate amounts of fuel - calories from fats, carbs, and proteins. Because there is adequate fuel, but an inability to turn that fuel into energy, we can say that ***fat gain is ultimately a problem of turning fuel into energy.***

I'll discuss this more in a bit, but there are also different ways of producing energy, and while some studies show that obese people burn more calories per day than thin people, they're actually burning those calories through a stress metabolism which is creating harmful metabolic by-products and perpetuating their metabolic dysfunction even further.

I want to illustrate this concept with a few scenario examples, to help it sink in...

Scenario #1: The Typical Overweight Person:

In this scenario, we're looking at the classic overweight man or woman. Their cells have low energy flow, but there is a surplus of fuel coming into the system. This individual is not able to convert this fuel into energy that the cells can use (for reasons I will discuss later, one of which being the actual quality of the fuel they've provided to their system), and therefore this fuel gets stored as "excess" body fat tissue.

Scenario #2: The Typical Overweight Person Goes On A Traditional "Diet":

In this scenario, we have the typical overweight person from scenario #1 again, however in this case, they go on a "diet" and start consuming fewer calories than before. In fact, now they're consuming the exact same amount of calories that their cells are able to use as energy. At first, they will stop storing excess fat, since now their cells are translating this fuel into energy that can flow through their body. However, since they never addressed the original problem (ie. the fact that their cells are in a low energy state), any prolonged period of eating calories at this low level may add further distress on the cellular functioning, lowering the metabolic rate even further.

This is also very common for overweight individuals, and typically ends in frustration and a "rebound" along the pendulum of compensation.

The ironic thing is this: most people think the calories are the sole issue, when in fact, it's more about your cellular capability to handle the translation of the fuel into cellular energy available for use in the body. This is one of the common pitfalls people step into when they start making arguments about how diets don't work for them, or how "calories don't matter" because when they dropped calories they didn't lose weight. They focus on the wrong thing, chiefly out of ignorance.

Scenario #3: The Balanced Thermo Person:

In this scenario, we have a person who is consuming a lot of fuel but who is also able to turn all of that fuel into energy within the cells. This person may be consuming the same amount of fuel as the person in scenario 1, but they won't be storing fat because everything they eat gets used by their cells. What's more, this person will be producing a ton of energy within their cells, allowing them to easily meet their energy needs for survival functions, and have plenty of energy for their thriving functions like growth and maintenance. This person will likely experience a shift in body composition without a change in weight, as their body will naturally have less of a reason to store fat in the first place, and will begin using that fat energy for growth and maintenance purposes (like creating hormones and important enzymes).

Scenario #4: Person In Fat Loss Phase Of The Thermo Diet:

Finally, in this scenario, we have the person who is able to create energy freely from fuel, and they're consuming less fuel than their body needs each day. This person will be easily and readily tapping into their fat stores for fuel, since their cells will be converting any fuel they get into energy, and not getting enough fuel from food. While this sounds like the ideal situation for fat loss, consuming too few calories over time will eventually slow down your cells' ability to produce energy, **so the ideal is really to hover between scenarios 3 and 4.** This will allow you to lose fat while balancing it with maintaining cellular energy production from fuel sources.

So, to wrap up the important concepts around bioenergetics that you need to understand, I will summarize this as follows...

Bioenergetics is the truth that your biology is dependent on the flow of energy throughout its systems. This is supported as foundational scientific fact, and illustrated through many cellular reactions.

Most people have an energy problem.

The flow of energy through their body is impaired by "blockers.". This is the culprit of disease and any biological dysfunction. Nearly everyone, through ignorance and the spread of misinformation, is confused and focused on entirely the wrong things.

As our population continues to focus on the wrong things, rates of autoimmune diseases, cancers, and obesity continue to rise to staggering heights. Record heights. Something's terribly wrong with the way we've been looking at our health, and now is the time to fix it.

The first step toward fixing your health, is to understand the idea of coherence and not only how it applies to your cellular functioning, but also how your cellular coherence effects, either positively or negatively, the functioning of your tissues, organs, and organ systems.

Coherence is the quality of forming a unified whole.

Your body seeks coherence naturally, without you having to think about it. However, while it may prefer to find coherence based on positive, health-giving factors, if you continually influence it in a negative way, with negative inputs, then it will develop coherence in the negative state. This is evident when disease arises in the body, however this negative coherence has many other warning signs, from bloating, inflammation, fatigue, brain fog, poor libido, sexual dysfunction, poor sleep, and so forth.

As we all learned in elementary school science class, your mitochondria are responsible for facilitating the energy flow in the body, and when cells begin to allow energy to flow in a healthy, productive way, they produce more signals to other cells to let them know what they are doing.

This is crucial because for all of the cells to organize themselves into one coherent organism up the chain of tissues, organs, organ systems, and ultimately, *you*, they need to work in concert with each other. The system would become disorganized and ineffective if certain cells were behaving completely independently of other cells.

These communication systems within the body work in many different ways, on different levels, and in multiple directions, and the messengers including everything from hormones, to neurotransmitters, to electrolytes, to metabolic by-products.

For example, when cells produce energy from glucose using their mitochondria, they produce a lot of energy and a lot of carbon dioxide, CO2. But when they produce energy in an inefficient way due to stress factors, they produce far less energy, and lactic acid instead of carbon dioxide.

Carbon dioxide is a signal to all levels of your body that cells are producing energy via the efficient "respiration" pathways, and that encourages others cells to do the same. This positive acceleration of metabolism is moderated by the lactic acid signal, which signals to all levels of your body that cells are producing energy via the inefficient "glycolytic" pathways, and again, that encourages other cells to do the same thing in order to maintain coherence.

A good way to think of this is that each level of your body is simply a connection of similar structures that are social with one another. Your cells are social with other cells, your tissues are social with other tissues, and your organs are social with other organs - just like you are social with other people.

If you were to walk into a room to find all of your friends somber, quiet, and depressed, you would pick up on these signals and it would discourage you from being gregarious, loud, and overly chipper.

These signals that your friends are emitting help you to read the context of the social environment you are in so that you can connect as a part of something bigger - the social group that you and your friends make up, just like the signals your cells produce are helping the other cells to read the context of the *chemical environment* they are in so that they can connect as a part of something bigger - the tissue that they make up.

Your cells are constantly *reading the environment* to gain an understanding of what the other cells are doing, but they are also emitting their own signals at the same time, which help play into the collective environment.

To go back to our previous analogy, if your group of friends were all somber, you would pick up on this cue and know not to act outrageously. But at the same time, you are also sending out a signal that they are picking up on, and if you act in a way that brightens each person's mood, then you can help to improve the collective mood of the group.

Your cells are behaving the same way, constantly reading the environment from the other cells, while also exercising their own influence over the collective.

But the environment is not *only* made up of what other cells are doing - wider and more far-reaching signals from higher levels of organization have a big impact on the collective groups of cells as well as on the individual level.

The 5 Laws Of The Thermo Diet

"A given structure makes possible a certain level of useful energy, and adequate energy makes possible the maintenance of structure, and the advance to a higher and more efficient structural level." - Dr. Ray Peat PhD.

At its core, the Thermo Diet, and the Commandments of Nutrition outlined in detail inside this book, are based on a solid foundation of unwavering Laws that hold true throughout every organism.

This is part of what makes the Thermo Diet so powerful - it's built on top of concepts that hold true throughout all of nature, of which humans are not exempt.

These Laws define the way systems work at every level, from the cells, up to the tissues, to the organs, and then even the interaction between organs, known as the *organ systems.*

Ultimately, this all leads to the Laws that define how YOU function, since your body is a collection of organ systems, which are each a collection of organs, which are each a collection of tissue, which are each a collection of cells.

Things become much clearer when we look at how these Laws apply to individual cells, as long as we remember the bigger picture, and connect the dots between individual cells and the whole organism that is you. By looking at how individual cells work, we can gain a better understanding of their organization on each level, and ultimately allow us to see what practical steps we can take to impact all of our cells, which make up our entire body.

What's more, these Laws are so simple that you'll likely find yourself nodding along, thinking "of course that's true" as we dive into them - the Truth of these Laws is powerful, yet obvious.

With that, there are 5 specific Laws that define the basis of the Thermo Diet and cellular optimization.

Law #1: More Energy Flow Is Better Than Less

Energy is a resource, just like any other resource, and the more resources you have, the better you function and the more you can do.

When resources are scarce - in any situation - you have to prioritize what you will use those resources for, in order to make sure your necessities are covered.

For example, you wouldn't want to spend your paycheck on a vacation when you need that money to pay rent. Rent is important for your survival, and therefore needs to be paid first before you spend money (aka the "resource") on "thriving" things like going on a vacation.

The same is true on a cellular level.

Cells produce energy by turning carbs and fats into molecules of "ATP" (or adenosine triphosphate). This is the basic energy storage unit for cells, and more ATP means more energy readily available.

Therefore, you can view the production of ATP like you would view your income, where the amount of ATP your cells produce is equivalent to the size of your paycheck.

Few people would argue that a larger paycheck is a bad thing, since you'll now have more resources to not only pay for your necessities, but now enjoy higher things like vacations, luxuries, and charity. You no longer stress over whether or not you can pay for things important to your survival, like utility bills and rent/mortgage, since you're no longer in a state of scarcity, but rather a state of abundance.

Just like you, your cells have survival functions that must be "paid for" before higher functions like growth and maintenance can come into play. ATP is the currency your cells spend on these functions, and the more ATP your cells can create and use, the more energy they have to spend on not only the survival functions, but the thriving functions as well, which is where the essence to radiating health exists.

When cells are in a higher energetic state, they are stronger and more capable of handling stresses. They not only have enough energy to keep you alive, but also to increase the quality of your life.

Law #2: Energy Is Flow, Change, & Transition

While ATP is the storage form of energy for your cells, it's crucial to realize that they are not actual energy in and of themselves - the energy is released when your cells break a phosphate group off of ATP, converting it to ADP (adenosine diphosphate, with only two phosphates instead of three).

That's because energy cannot be stagnant - it cannot stay still. Energy, by definition, is movement, transition, change... energy is flow.

Therefore, a crucial aspect of cellular energy is not simply having high ATP levels, but rather a high use of ATP - breaking it down for energy - alongside a high replenishment of ATP - restoring ATP through the metabolism of carbohydrates and fats.

This provides a higher flow or *flux*, which means that your cells are actually using a lot of energy while simultaneously replenishing that energy.

Similar to money, ATP doesn't necessarily help you if you don't use it. A million dollars in a bank account that you can never access is useless to you, because it's the spending - or *flow* - of money that matters, not simply the possession of it.

Even if you were allowed to spend $10 per month from that million dollar bank account, you still wouldn't get more value than that $10.

But if you're spending a lot of money while simultaneously making a lot of money, then you get all the value in your life that comes using money for things, while continually replenishing it to keep getting that value. The total amount you have matters much less than the use and replenishment of it.

In your cells, using ATP for energy allows them to grow, maintain, heal, restore, and ultimately, thrive, and the constant replenishment of that ATP ensures that this thriving continues.

On the other hand, maintaining the same constant level of ATP in your cells, but using it slower and replenishing it slower (aka, a slower flow), will not give you as much benefit because you're using less energy.

So in order to increase energy in the cell, you need to increase the flow of processes through the cell.

It's the *movement* through the cell that is the underlying aspect that drives the function and structure and improves its health.

Law #3: How You Produce Energy Flow Matters

While producing a greater flow of energy is important, how you produce that energy flow is also important, primarily because the metabolic by-products created will encourage either higher or lower energy production systemically, shifting the overall way cells act.

In other words, if you produce a lot of energy in a way that triggers slower energy production, you won't continue producing high levels of energy in the long-term. The negative coherence you're actively creating will eventually lower the energy flow of your entire system.

There are two main ways your cells produce energy: from glucose or fatty acids.

Another way to think about this is to envision two main energy production pathways in the body. One of these pathways is organized in a manner that makes up the "healthy metabolism," including beneficial metabolic by-products. This healthy metabolism pathway has an abundant energy flow and is highly efficient. This is the glucose metabolism.

The other pathway is considered the "stress metabolism," a pathway characteristic of inefficient energy produced from a state of lack of the abundant preferred energy in the healthy metabolism pathway. This stress metabolism is a survival mechanism, keeping the organism alive long enough for it to find additional fuel sources to kickstart the healthy metabolism again. It should be a last resort for the body when energy needs aren't otherwise met. This is the fatty acid metabolism.

Hopefully now you can easily envision the different ways of energy production and flow in the body. Many people fall into the *oversimplification trap* of measuring their metabolic health based solely on total energy burned. The pathway used for this energy production and flow is of paramount importance and cannot be overlooked!

Just measuring the total energy output from a person throughout a day may give you a "total energy burn number" that most people blanketly associate as "metabolism", but in Truth, the way this energy is produced in paramount to your overall health and well-being, not to mention your fat loss efforts.

For example, many obese people may burn more calories per day than a thin person, but you can almost guarantee they have higher levels of adrenaline, cortisol, and lactic acid - hallmarks of the stress metabolism, and likely part of the reason why they're obese.

We'll dive deeper into more of the science behind the difference between the healthy metabolism and the stress metabolism in this book, but for now it's only important to realize that the healthy metabolism is responsible for creating more energy and a higher flow of energy, while the stress metabolism does just the opposite.

Law #4: Like Attracts Like - The Way You Produce Energy Creates More Of The Same

When your cells produce energy via the healthy metabolism, good by-products are produced that encourage other cells to produce more energy from the healthy metabolism as well.

On the other hand, the stress metabolism encourages less energy production overall, and more energy to be produced from the stress metabolism.

All of this to say that one of the core laws of the universe - that like attracts like - applies to health, metabolism, and weight loss, too.

The idea behind this is that cause and effect in the body actually works in both directions - something can cause an effect, but that effect is causing the first thing as well, at the same time. We can call this a "two-way street" or more scientifically, a *feedback loop.*

All this means is that because everything works within loops in your body, you can't say that one thing causes another, but that both things are causing each other in a cycle.

When it comes to metabolism, the major point to grasp is that producing energy via the healthy metabolism will create a higher energetic state within the cell along with healthier metabolic by-products. This higher energy state and these healthier metabolic by-products will then create a higher level of the healthy metabolism, spurring on an upward spiral of health, regeneration. The same can work in reverse with the stress metabolism, causing a downward spiral of health, degeneration.

Our job then, if we're looking to achieve an acceleration upwards towards the state of radiating health, is to encourage an increase in healthy metabolism, energy state, and healthy metabolic by-products, while discouraging the stress metabolism, lower energy states, and stressful metabolic by-products.

Law #5: Biological Rhythm Determines Default Metabolism

Once the energetic state, flux, and pathway of energy production have been set for a while, it becomes entrained to the cell as it's default mode, which is changeable only through deliberate and consistent efforts.

Once your cells have been operating in a certain way for some time, they begin to become entrained into a rhythm based on that way they're operating.

This is the basic idea of a *setpoint* in the body, which is often used when describing body weight regulation, but applies to all areas in your body.

This connects to the previous Law, because as a certain way of producing energy continues to encourage the cells to continue creating energy in that way, over time the collective context within your body will shift away from any other methods of energy creation and towards stability in whatever way is in focus.

For the sake of explaining this concept, let's imagine an organism that has 10 cells in its body that are all producing energy in a poor way. If 1 of those cells begins to produce energy in a better way, it will produce by-products and other chemical signals to tell the other cells what it's doing.

If the other 9 cells are producing energy in a poor way and sending out signals as well, then the one cell will have a hard time continuing to produce energy in the healthy way, because it's constantly being told that all the other cells aren't producing energy that way, and the survival of the organism is dependent on all the cells working together.

Another way to say this is that 90% of the total organism's energy is being created in a poor way, and 10% is being created in a healthy way, which means that each individual cell is getting a 90/10 signal, encouraging them to produce 90% of their energy in a poor way and 10% in a good way.

Because each cell is receiving this signal, the cells will begin to shift their energy production to match the total average, assuming it remains at a 90/10 split. This means that all the cells producing energy in a poor way will begin producing 10% of their energy in a good way, while the cell producing all its energy in the good way will shift to producing 90% of its energy in the poor way.

Now if you are able to change conditions to improve the function of the cells so that 50% are producing energy in a good way, then that signal will get locked into the biological rhythm, and the cells will all start producing 50% of their energy the good way, and 50% the poor way.

While individual cells don't completely change their energy production in the way described, the changing of internal conditions does slowly shift the way cells produce energy, and once that becomes stable through all of the cells producing energy in the same way and communicating that to each other, then a new baseline is created.

Once this new baseline is created, changing conditions positively or negatively will cause a deviation in the way the cells behave, but always with a tendency to return to the baseline, since that has been established and solidified through the communicative network between cells. Only after the internal conditions are changed for long enough for the cells to all begin operating differently, and therefore communicating differently, can a new baseline be established.

This is the basis of how metabolic derangement and obesity happens in the first place, as some internal condition that encourages poor energy production is present for long enough to cause all of the cells to become entrained to this way of operating, setting a new, lower baseline.

Believe it or not, this is actually the way that *inherited health* works, as your cells are entrained based on conditions in the womb, based on your mother's level of health and the interaction between your genes and that environment.

You're born at a certain baseline based on this interaction of the environment in the womb and your genes, which is the reason some people seemed to have won the genetic lottery while others are born with poor health out of the gate.

However, it's important to recognize the power we hold in this understanding - no matter where your baseline currently is or even where it was when you were born, you have the ability to improve the internal conditions and raise that baseline. No one is doomed to poor health simply because of genes; in fact, your genes interact with your environment so strongly that you can change genetic expression by changing your environment strongly enough.

Similarly, no one is doomed to poor health because of previous health conditions - you are capable of improving your health in this present moment by taking the right steps forward, to change your internal environment and default metabolism.

These Laws Will Always Ring True

Because the universe exhibits the concepts of infinity in all aspects, with infinite smaller fractals and and infinite larger fractals of the same thing, we can assume that these Laws apply to that which is smaller than the cell, and that which is larger than a single person (a community, a nation, or even the entire species, and so forth).

An important distinction between the analogy of money to ATP in your cells is that unlike money, ATP has very limited storage, and is more reliant on its rate of production to maintain high energy levels.

It's important to realize that ATP isn't the actual energy your cells use. Instead, when your cells' convert ATP into ADP, energy is then *released* and used by the cell.

As I mentioned above, ATP is not energy in and of itself - it is only when your cells break a phosphate group off of ATP, converting it to ADP, that energy is released.

And since it's the *use of energy* that is important, a higher flow both in and out results in a higher *use* of the energy, and therefore a more abundant state of thriving, versus a scarce state of survival.

It also may be helpful to picture a river. A river with an extremely slow current will build up algae and waste, dirtying the water, while a fast moving river will stay clean and crisp.

Secrets Of A Healthy Metabolism

If you've ever had difficulty losing fat despite doing everything "right" and eating less food like you've been told, then the stress metabolism is at play.

In fact, most people and almost every fat loss diet out there relies on using the stress metabolism to lose weight, which only results in long-term metabolic derangements and a slower metabolism.

Once someone has used the stress metabolism too much for weight loss, it stops working, and despite your best efforts, the weight just doesn't come off. The solution, as I'm laying out in this book, is to restore healthy metabolic functioning, and let that improved metabolism raise your level of health so that your body naturally wants to lose weight, rather than trying to force it through stress.

Of course this offers many more advantages as well, like

effortless results, a better quality of life, and a higher enjoyment of food.

The Survive-Thrive Scale

The best way to understand how your body functions based on the different types of metabolism is by looking at what I call the *Survive-Thrive Scale.*

This is a spectrum that shows the different levels your body might be at, as a result of the type of metabolism it consistently uses, along with other individual factors.

On the high side of the spectrum, we have the thrive side.

This is where your body is in peak health, functioning at its highest evolutionary potential, fueling your life, well-being, and joy.

And of course, in this state, fat loss is incredibly easy. Your body is in an abundant state and has no need to hold onto fat. It's also not bogged down by toxins as your liver is easily capable of quickly processing and excreting any toxins you might be exposed to.

This state is characterized by high thyroid function and low adrenaline, as all the cells in your body are operating off of the healthy, oxidative metabolism, producing those healthy by-products like carbon dioxide.

In this state, your body is easily able to handle stress, and is consistently recovering and replenishing more than it is facing stressors, leading to a positive stress balance.

As we move down the scale, we slip into a state where health begins to decline, but not to an excessive level. Here, fat loss is difficult and you have to be very strict with your food intake and micromanage your calorie count in order to see progress.

This state is characterized by an increase in adrenaline and a decrease in thyroid function, as your body is beginning to rely more and more on the stress metabolism. Because thyroid function has declined, your body is now relying on adrenaline to signal cells to quickly and inefficiently produce energy, producing the negative by-products that signal lower and lower healthy metabolism, like lactic acid.

At the same time, your body is now more resistant to adrenaline, and has to pump out a lot more of it to get the increase in energy it's looking for. In fact, towards the end of the Minnesota Starvation Experiment, they found that injecting pure adrenaline into the subjects had hardly any effects at all because of how desensitized to it they had become.

This state is also where your body is facing a stressor, which is why it's using the stress metabolism and pumping out more adrenaline in order to produce the energy it needs.

Finally, on the low end we have the survival side.

This is characterized by low energy, poor skin/hair/nail quality, bad sleep, impotence, and brain fog - all around poor health. In this part of the scale, fat loss is basically impossible, and no matter how much you restrict caloric intake, you seem to be "stuck" with your fat loss efforts.

This state is characterized by both low thyroid function AND low adrenaline, as your body has shifted into pure survival mode, reducing your energy output and metabolism as low as possible while storing any food it can as fat for protection.

Your adrenal glands have been exhausted from pumping out so much adrenaline, that now they "give up" and no longer produce much adrenaline.*

**This is a state that many people call "Adrenal Fatigue", and while adrenaline is low, it's really a problem of low thyroid and metabolic function.*

This is the stage where you've exhausted your body's ability to face the stress, and now it's simply giving up and doing it's best to survive.

While this might sound pretty grim, it's a reality that many people are living everyday, and are often told is normal.

Not only is the survival state of health not normal (or pleasant, or productive), but even the middle of the scale - where the majority of people exist - is not normal.

You were meant to live in the thrive state, with exceptional and enjoyable health, where fat loss is simple and your level of health is visible and attractive as it radiates from your skin.

How To Move Up The Survive-Thrive Scale

So the question now becomes, how do you move up and down the scale? What causes the changes that lead your body to recalibrate at different points?

It all comes down to your *Net Stress Balance*, or NSB, in any given period of time.

If your NSB is positive for a 24-hour period, then you will move up the scale in proportion to the level of net positive you were in.

In other words, your movement up the scale depends on how big your positive NSB is, and how long you maintain it. Ideally, you want to be in a positive NSB for most of the time in order to continually allow your health to float back up to its natural, high level of health on the thrive side of the scale.

Your Net Stress Balance is just what it sounds like - the overall balance between stressors that negatively affect your body, and recovery factors that help heal and restore your body.

I call these stressors that negatively affect your body *blockers*, as they block your body's natural tendency to raise towards the thrive side of the scale, and pull it down towards the survival side.

These are things you want to avoid.

On the other hand, there are certain things that promote recovery and healing, and increase the healthy metabolism in cells, which will help your body move up towards the thrive side of the scale.

I call these healing factors *activators,* as they activate your body's natural recovery processes, aiding in its rise towards that vibrant, thriving state.

Finally, there are certain factors that improve your NSB when in balance, which lower your NSB when too low or too high.

I call these factors *balancers,* as they're crucial for your health, but must not be over or under done. These include stressors that can make your body more resilient once your body has recovered from them, like exercise.

When combining all of these, if we want to promote a more positive NSB, we want to add as many activators as we can into our lives, while avoiding the blockers, and keeping the balancers at the right levels.

If we continue to do this for enough time, we'll maintain that positive NSB for long enough to trigger a movement of our body up the Survive-Thrive Scale, and see noticeable and tangible changes in our bodies, including faster fat loss and a leaner body composition.

Activators, Blockers, and Balancers

Now it's time to discuss activators, blockers and balancers. These are all very important concepts to understand in the context of approaching the Thermo Diet in a way that's going to make you successful.

Blockers

Blockers are things that you've introduced into your life, starting from when you were a kid all the way through your teenage years, which eventually start to cause stress on your body.

This is typically in the form of physiological stress, which is free radical damage to your body. This results in an inflammatory response of some type. Eventually, not only your immune system but also your endocrine system becomes compromised, and you start to degrade into a disease state.

This happens through the reinforcement of negative coherence. As you continue to introduce blockers into your body over and over and over again, you start to reinforce this negative coherence and eventually have a diseased body.

Activators

Activators are the opposite of that.

Activators are things that you can introduce into your body that are going to fight against the free radical stress and the free radical damage in the body. By doing so, they're going to really help balance your health and keep you in a state of good health. They're going to bring you back toward that Thermo State whereas blockers are taking you away from the Thermo State.

Activators are bringing you back into that state of perfect health. The end goal is to decrease the amount of blockers in your life and increase the amount of activators in your life – on a daily basis.

Balancers

Balancers are things that are somewhat in the middle. They aren't as cut and dry as blockers and activators, which are inherently very clear (it's clear that a blocker is bad and an activator is good).

With balancers, you need to have a bit more discretion and information. What we're going to do is look at the reality and practicality of the balancers.

For example, a balancer would be protein consumption. Carbs and fats clearly will fit into other categories whereas with protein consumption, you can over consume proteins with unfavorable amino acid makeups to the point where it is detrimental. You could also under consume protein to the point where it's detrimental.

Chapter 5 is entirely focused on the concept of protein consumption as a balancer, and how to determine your ideal protein intake to best support your health goals.

This is why it's important to be clear on the balancers, which is something we'll get into more detail on in that section.

Those are the three things that we're going to be focusing on throughout the book in some form or another. Specifically, we'll look at:

- **Blockers** – things that are getting in the way of optimal health and taking you away from thermo
- **Activators** – things that you should be introducing into your body to help bring you back toward the Thermo State, and
- **Balancers** –things that are going to help balance your health and to help with a stress cycle, the survival-thrive scale and help with the eustress and distress

In designing the thinking tools around this book, and the simple philosophy laid out inside it, I firmly believe this structure to be the easiest way to grasp the information, and a great tool for you to use to filter recommendations and make good choices for your health.

Throughout the book I will classify the recommendations using these terms.

Let's get into the details...

CHAPTER ONE

DON'T BE DEFICIENT

THE LAW OF MICRONUTRIENTS

Modern medical education does not focus on the human body's absolute need for vitamins, minerals, and amino acids to fuel every hormonal, metabolic, and enzymatic process required for basic living requirements. Because of this, the vital importance of nutrients has completely escaped the public's attention. Meanwhile, the modern food supply, coupled with mass confusion around dieting habits, fad diets, and commercial farming practices has led to widespread population-level micronutrient deficiencies across the world. These deficiencies cause most health problems, from sexual dysfunction, to metabolic disorders, thyroid, brain, and circulation disorders, and even hair loss, and thanks to recent scientific and entrepreneurial developments, can be easily corrected with affordable, accessible in-home testing and supplementation protocols with a focus on bioavailability and gut health. Determine your deficiencies, so you can quickly correct them to restore your body back to homeostatic functioning.

"If it wasn't for zinc, D3, and magnesium, I'd be dead or in prison right now - they saved my fucking life," Jeff tells me.

Jeff (name changed at his request for anonymity, but he's a very real person), has a story not unlike many other people I've talked to over the years, albeit his may be a little more extreme than most.

At the heart of his journey lies drug use, all pharmaceutical and other legal drugs, misinformed doctors, and one important blood test that completely changed everything. In fact, it's not unlike my own story. The pattern is common in this day and age. You might see some of your own story in this too.

As a child, Jeff was plagued with unexplained skin rashes, sore muscles, and bad mood swings. It wasn't until he was in his 20's before he found out why, since childhood he had experienced these issues.

When Jeff was a teenager, like most kids his age, he discovered alcohol. Drinking became a pastime, something he used for recreation and competition with his buddies. It quickly turned into a form of self-medication to escape the pains of daily life. When he started working in a hydraulics plant, he got a prescription from the family doctor for adderall, using amphetamines as a strong upper to balance out the depressant effects of his nightly drinking, helping him get up in the morning and stay alert on a demanding job.

"This brought on its own series of problems," he said.

His mood swings got worse. He started street fighting. Then, within a 6 month time period, Jeff's father and his girlfriend both committed suicide. To cope with the trauma, he saw a doctor who prescribed him an antidepressant and the antipsychotic drug Seroquel, to help him fall asleep.

"So I was just pumping my body with so much trash just to get out of bed and function and then I needed to bring myself down at the end of the day," he tells me.

Soon, he started experiencing issues with erectile dysfunction. His libido completely disappeared.

This is when the warning bells started to ring.

Jeff stopped taking the antidepressant and Seroquel, and started looking for a different kind of doctor, someone he could trust to give him some real facts about how to turn his health around.

He found a doctor who came highly recommended in an affluent area of Australia, and after a 90 minute appointment explaining his history she ordered him a blood panel to measure his micronutrient levels. She recognized some patterns in his behavior that have been observed as signs of key deficiencies, especially with respect to mental health, by researchers in the field of nutrient studies, like the alcohol abuse, rashes, and mood swings.

The blood test results showed massively high levels of copper in Jeff's blood, along with some glaring deficiencies in zinc, magnesium, Vitamin D, and the B vitamins.

She immediately put Jeff on a high daily dose of zinc picolinate, D3, B vitamins, and magnesium powder. After about 3 months of *"feeling pretty average with the supplements"* Jeff experienced a massive breakthrough that this doctor had told him would be coming... He finally passed the copper out of his body.

"I remember it was Christmas at my mums," he explained. *"I had curled up in one of the downstairs bedrooms; I had a terrible stomach ache and had to sit on the toilet for a while. What came out was bright orange turds. The doctor told me this was the copper passing out of my body."*

After that day, Jeff started to feel better and better every day. He stayed on his daily supplement regimen and within months he ditched all drugs he was using and massively cut down on his alcohol intake. He went from daily binge drinking for a decade to *"only having 12 beers this year."*

He says he now *"feels 100x better than when [he] was growing up."* Fixing his deficiencies helped clear away childhood health issues too.

And best of all, Jeff's *"crippling depression is now completely gone!"* He used to stay home alone to avoid people, but now he works as a successful project manager in a construction company and spends most of his day (willingly) socializing and coordinating large scale projects with his peers. He's also taken his experience and is now helping his family members. Recently he helped his brother get off his antidepressants and pursue a natural nutrient based therapy for depression.

In his words, *"I hate to think about how many people out there can be happy and anxiety-free and feel great in their life but are stuck on these pharmaceuticals the doctors are pumping them full of which is doing nothing but putting a wet blanket over their symptoms."*

So why doesn't the general public know about the importance of nutrients, and the devastating effect of nutrient deficiencies on their health?

One of the main reasons is the lack of nutrition education in medical schools. A lagging medical school curriculum with almost zero focus on nutrition remains the societal chokepoint for mass awareness around nutrients, mainly due to the fact that a majority of the population still looks to medical doctors for solutions to their health problems. This appeal to authority will no longer serve us in the development of our understanding of human health, and the evidence only gets clearer and clearer that it, to this point, has done nothing but send us in the wrong direction.

This sentiment has begun to shift slightly over the past decade due to the faster spread of information over the internet, and ability to gain access to legitimate scientific literature databases.

However, not every person who reads, or spreads, information is necessarily qualified to accurately disseminate its meaning, and therefore the spread of misinformation has also simultaneously become easier, leaving people more confused than ever about the right way to eat for health, and leaving them vulnerable to predatory marketing and propaganda.

Governing medical bodies have analyzed and surveyed medical school curriculums for decades. All surveys have come to similar conclusions about the inadequacy of nutrition education, such as "the amount of nutrition education in medical schools remains inadequate,"[1] and "the amount of nutrition education US medical students receive continues to be inadequate,"[2] with that specific 2010 study citing the fact that only 26 medical schools in the US (out of the 127 accredited US medical schools) required a dedicated nutrition course during the entire curriculum.

The fact that so few medical schools actually require nutrition training is also concerning when coupled with the finding that a declining number of medical students are actually interested in learning anything about nutrition at all.[3] A review in 2011 referenced the cause of this decline in interest as potentially being related to the fact that, since the 1950s, medical students have all carried a similar sentiment that nutrition education in medical school is inadequate, similar to the studies cited previously. Another more recent study in 2017[4] in the journal Family Medicine found the exact same thing: doctors across the board think that nutrition education is poorly integrated into the medical school curriculum. "They witnessed little nutrition counseling during shadowing experiences, and the nutrition information imparted was often outdated or incorrect." And medical students entering residency programs "appear to be deficient in basic nutritional knowledge."[5]

When you combine a lack of trust in the quality of the education itself, paired with no improvement in curriculum (or even a requirement to learn nutrition basics in most US medical schools), it seems perfectly reasonable to understand why fewer and fewer doctors are even interested in learning anything about nutrition during their expensive schooling. After all, why would you want to spend thousands of dollars taking course material that your peers since the 1950s, and even governing medical organizations, all deem "inadequate."

The dissatisfaction with medical school nutrition education is not reserved for institutions in the United States, however, with another study[6] in the Canadian Journal of Applied Physiology, Nutrition, and Metabolism demonstrating an average score of 4.7 for Canadian medical students' sentiments about the quality of their nutrition education on a scale of 1 to 10 (with 1 being immense dissatisfaction and 10 being satisfaction). Of the students surveyed, 87.3% of them believed that their curriculum should dedicate more time to nutrition education, referencing the fact that most of the medical students were "uncomfortable discussing the role of nutrition in the treatment of disease and nutrient requirements across the lifecycle."

According to data from the National Health and Nutrition

Examination Survey (NHANES) in the United States,[7, 8, 9, 10]

- More than 2 in 3 adults are considered to be overweight or obese, which is classified as at or above the 85th percentile on the CDC growth charts.
- More than 1 in 3 adults are obese, which is at or above the 95th percentile on the CDC growth charts.
- About 1 in 13 adults were considered extremely obese, which is at or above 120% of the 95th percentile on the CDC growth charts.
- About 1 in 6 children and adolescents ages 2 to 19 are obese.

There is little doubt that overweight and obesity remains an escalating epidemic, at least in the US, however medical doctors, according to a recent 2017 study[11] in the medical Journal of Health Promotion Practice, still remain under pressure from "widespread expectations that primary care physicians counsel their overweight and obese patients" in nutrition despite the fact that very few medical school programs have given them what could be deemed as "adequate" training on the subject.

This, specifically, is a problem mostly because it is set up to fail both parties involved, the patient and the practitioner.

Obese and overweight patients go to see their doctors for specific weight-related health issues they're looking to solve, such as metabolic syndrome, Type 2 diabetes, high blood pressure, and sexual dysfunction, however with the doctors' lack of confidence in their nutritional schooling, very few of them ever give the patients any sort of lifestyle or nutrition-related advice for reversing their health issues naturally, instead opting to prescribe them pharmaceuticals for their ailments, a subject around which they have had much more training in the medical curriculum.

The pharmaceuticals tend to cause more issues than they solve, and neither the patient nor the practitioner ever actually get to the bottom of the true issue at hand, relegating the patient to a life of prescription drugs when that fate was most likely entirely unnecessary.

And even though as far back as 1995, with the release of the pivotal study[12] by Dr. Robert Kushner, MD where he recommended that nutrition and dietary counseling be carried out by all clinical physicians "in the delivery of preventative services by primary care physicians," very little has changed in the medical practice and the common clinic when it comes to actually giving patients nutritional advice. In fact, while primary care physicians still believe that it is within their realm of responsibility to provide nutritional counseling, many physicians still do not believe that their patients, specifically, would actually benefit from nutritional counseling,[13] a belief that is likely due to the lack of schooling around the subject of nutrition in the first place.

Accordingly, physicians frequently lack substantive nutrition knowledge and counseling skills necessary to successfully guide their patients.[14] A recent study found[15] that only 14% of resident physicians believed they were adequately trained to provide nutritional counseling.

So again, the crossroads we've come to at this point in time, is the fundamental mixture of a lack of nutritional education for our presiding physicians in a society who looks to physicians for guidance on their health. The physicians themselves have no confidence in the quality of nutritional education, if it is provided at all, in their medical school curriculum, and that coupled with the high expense of learning course material in medical school would seem like a reasonable decision to avoid the nutritional courses in the first place.

And while, according to CDC data, our population's health is spiraling out of control, the doctors we have been told to trust to fix our health are no more equipped to teach us how to eat than any other individual with a passing interest in nutrition.

So how do we get ourselves out of this mess?

First, we must decide to take control of our own health. Nobody cares about your health as much as you do. Stop abdicating your fate to someone else. The necessary first step to taking responsibility over your own body is to understand the basics of how the body works. You must understand micronutrients: the vitamins, minerals, amino acids, and gases that play vitally important roles in every process within the human body.

An understanding of your body's 'building blocks' reveals to you the fundamental truth, the key that will open the door to your perfect state of health. It's time we take a step back and look at the true Nature of the human body.

We've lost the forest for the trees; the time has come to open up a different way of thinking about your health, because like Sir Francis Bacon so eloquently stated in the Novum Organum,[16] the basis for the scientific method as we know it today,

> *"A quite different way must be opened up for the human intellect than men have known in the past, and new aids devised, so that the mind may exercise its right over nature."*

What Are Micronutrients?

The basic Oxford dictionary definition of a micronutrient is, "a chemical element or substance required in trace amounts for the normal growth and development of living organisms."[17]

More specifically, the term *micronutrient* encompasses vitamins, minerals, amino acids, and even gases such as oxygen and carbon dioxide that are required by the body of a living organism in order to properly carry out hormonal, metabolic, cellular, and neuronal functioning.

Micronutrients are not needed in as high raw amounts as macronutrients, by definition, so we tend to find the daily need for them between the microgram range up to just a few grams, depending on the micronutrient.

Despite this low raw material requirement, most people are massively deficient in key micronutrients their body needs. We will explore the reasons why in this chapter.

When the body is deficient in any important micronutrient, it has to compensate for the lack of the necessary material within the specific system that needs it by trying to find it elsewhere within the body.[18] For example, low calcium levels, also known as hypocalcemia,[19] which can be caused by a range of different things such as low thyroid function,[20] low dietary calcium intake,[21] kidney disorders,[22] and as a side effect of many pharmaceuticals,[23] will compromise the basic functioning of many important processes, especially neuronal communication,[24] since calcium is one of our main electrolytes, or electrically-charged minerals needed in cellular communication.

Over time, a chronic calcium deficiency can lead to disorders such as osteoporosis,[25] in this case because calcium is stored in the bones, and when the body needs it for basic neuronal functioning it will leech it from storage areas, like the bones, in order to attempt to maintain normal function.

Over time, this natural compensation mechanism can be deleterious to your health, developing into full-blown osteoporosis. This is precisely why it is not uncommon for people who develop bone disorders like osteoporosis to previously exhibit neurological dysfunction symptoms such as depression,[26] brain fog, soreness, and tingling in their extremities sometimes years before their osteoporosis diagnosis.

The body is trying to maintain normal functioning within the important systems like your nervous system and circulatory system, which have a higher priority to your survival than your bone health, however you can only escape the symptoms of this compensatory response for so long before it comes time to pay the piper.

This is why it is so important to pay close attention to your micronutrient levels, and monitor symptoms that may arise throughout your life, addressing them through the action steps I will outline in this book.

Before we dive further into this chapter I want to make sure to outline the exact micronutrients I will be referencing here in this book that you need to be aware of. Let's take a quick look at the amino acids, vitamins, and minerals that your body needs in order to run properly.

Amino Acids

All proteins in the body are made up of different chains of amino acids.[27] Proteins run along a spectrum in their complexity with direct relation to the number, order, and variety of amino acids that make up their structural chain.

The simplest way to picture an amino acid, and a structure that is common to all of them, is that amino acids are made up of a weak acid molecule group - containing carbon, oxygen, and hydrogen - attached to a strong acid group, containing nitrogen.

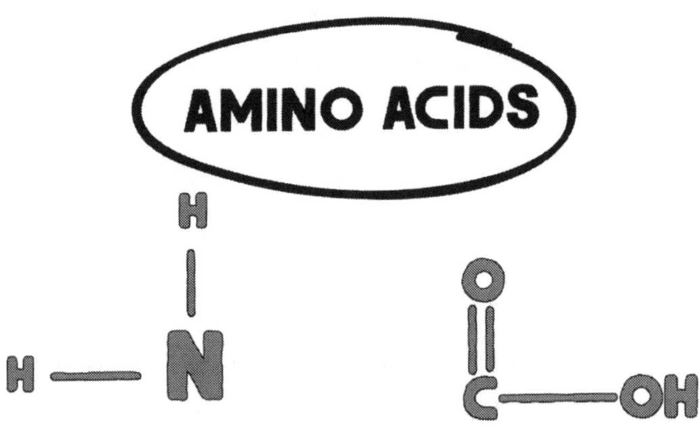

We typically group amino acids into two distinct types: essential amino acids and non-essential amino acids. Essential amino acids cannot be synthesized by the body and must be supplied by the diet.[28] They are:

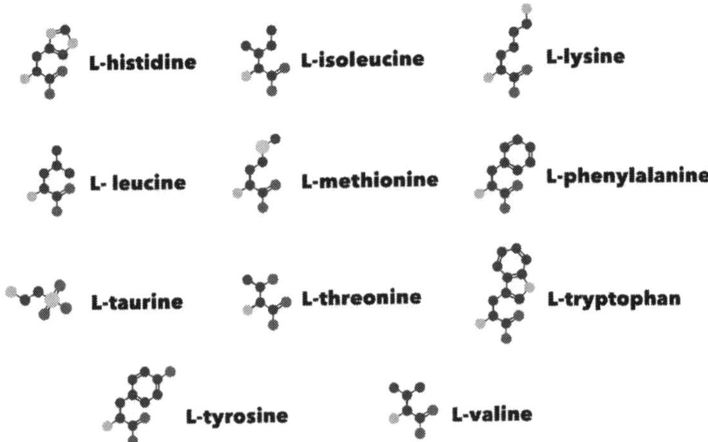

Non-essential amino acids can be synthesized by the body by combining two or more of the EAAs.[29] This combination would necessarily require adequate levels of the EAAs needed for the synthesis, however. NEAAs can become essential for the body during disease or disorder and stress because there is an increased need and/or breakdown of them. All stress states require more amino acids.[30] They are:

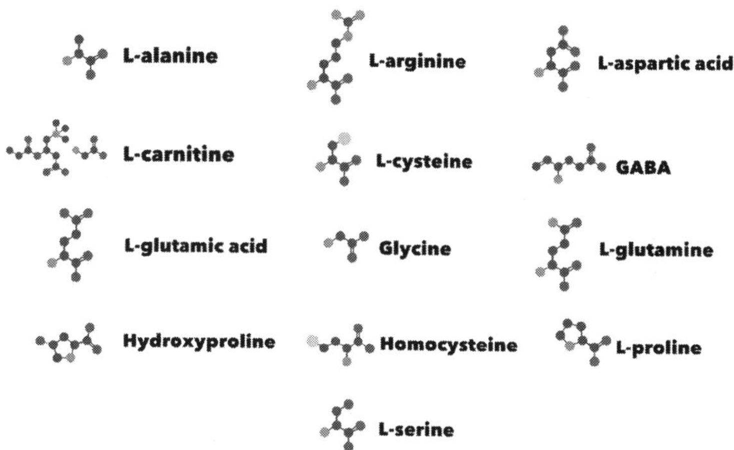

Vitamins

Vitamins are substances that the body needs for use as raw materials to fuel important metabolic processes, oftentimes by acting as cofactors.[31] For example, in the production of the neurotransmitter serotonin, the body requires the essential amino acid tryptophan,[32] and the final reaction step requires adequate availability of vitamin B6 as a cofactor in the process.[33] Without one of these nutrients, the process cannot happen correctly. Another example is the neurotransmitter norepinephrine which is produced in a process involving dopamine with copper as a cofactor.[34]

Vitamins are usually classified by their solubility, either

water-soluble or fat-soluble. The water soluble vitamins are the B vitamins and vitamin C.[35] Excess water soluble vitamins can be easily passed out of the body via urine. The fat soluble vitamins are vitamins A, D, E, and K. These must be more closely monitored as certain fat soluble vitamins can build up in tissue, such as vitamin A, leading to hypervitaminosis.[36]

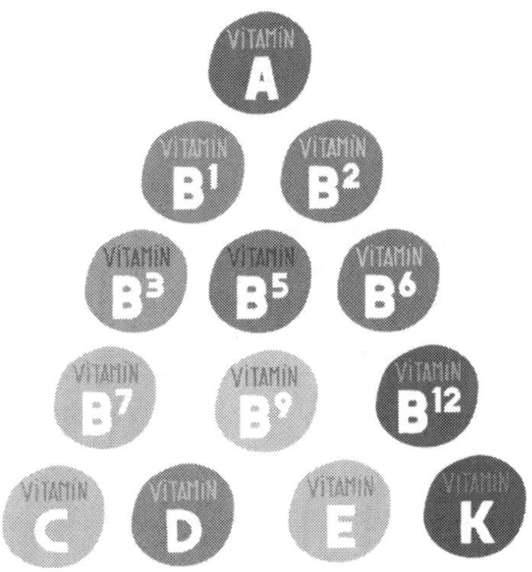

Minerals

While minerals, in general, are any solid inorganic natural substance, when people refer to the word "mineral" in the context of health, they usually mean two things: trace minerals and electrolytes. Both of which are absolutely essential in proper levels to the healthy functioning of your body.[37]

Trace minerals are critical minerals needed as building blocks for hundreds of different enzymes,[38] and are necessary for hormone functioning,[39] circulatory health,[40] can serve as antioxidants,[41] and are a requirement for healthy neurological functioning. They include:

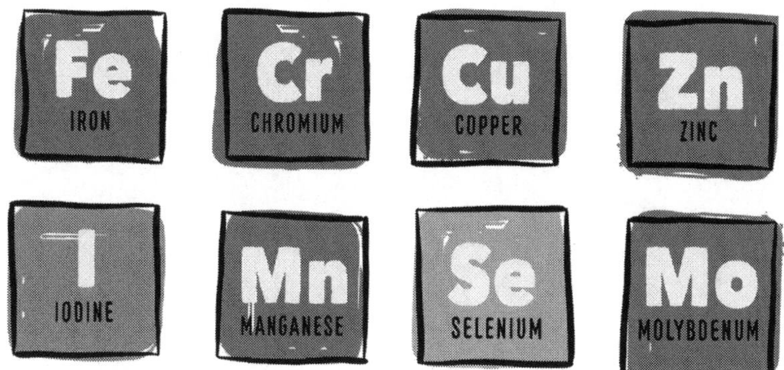

Electrolytes are minerals that when dissolved in the body's fluids create electrically charged ions.[42] Crack open any neuroscience or biochemistry textbook and you'll quickly realize how essential electrolytes are to literally every form of cellular communication in the body. Deficiency in any of the following nutrients can have a devastating effect on the way your cells operate and communicate with one another:

- Sodium[43]
- Potassium[44]
- Calcium[45]
- Magnesium[46]
- Phosphate[47]

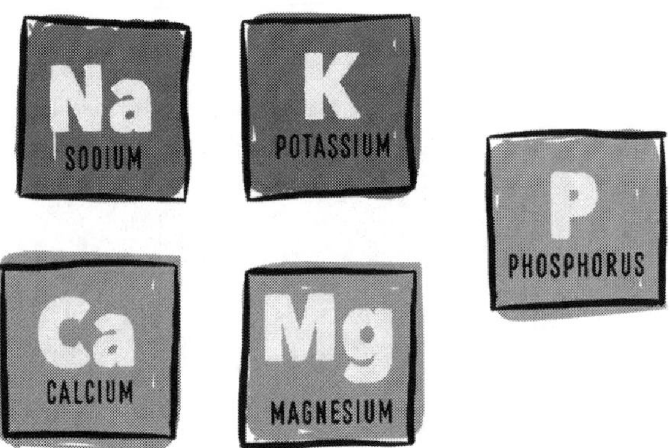

We will dive deep into the role of these electrolytes in aiding your optimal health throughout Chapter 2 (Eat More Salt).

What is a deficiency? And what causes them?

A micronutrient deficiency is quite literally a "lack" of one of the aforementioned nutrients that your body requires to fulfill its fundamental processes, like proper growth and metabolism.[48]

You might think, *"I eat healthy; I am not deficient in anything."*

You're wrong.

Statistically, half of the population of the entire world... yes the whole world... is deficient in multiple nutrients by the time they are 6 months old.[49] Between the ages of 6 months and 5 years old, this half of the world's children are deficient in iron, iodine, Vitamin A, folate, and zinc. These deficiencies cause, what the CDC refers to as, "devastating consequences."

Iron, for example, is essential in balanced levels in the body for cognitive and motor development from birth. One of the reasons that many children are iron deficient (along with other deficiencies) at or near birth is due to the deficiency of the mother.[50]

Anemia, low hemoglobin (a molecule in the blood responsible for transporting oxygen with a molecular structure containing four subunits each containing an iron atom bound to a heme group) in the blood, has been found to affect 38% of pregnant women globally.[51]

The iron deficiency is passed to the child at birth, and these prenatal deficiencies can also cause genetic and epigenetic expressions that become evident with age.[52]

Iodine, another extremely common prenatal deficiency, is a crucially important trace mineral needed for proper growth and development of the fetus, especially with relation to hormonal balance and brain development.[53]

Maternal iodine deficiency is *"recognized as the greatest cause of preventable mental impairment in the world,"* with 38 million newborn babies every year consequently at risk from iodine deficiency, and 18 million babies born yearly with iodine deficiency-caused mental impairment.[54]

It is estimated that worldwide, over 2 billion people do not consume adequate iodine to properly fuel their body's daily requirements.[55]

Vitamin A, a crucial fat-soluble vitamin necessary in the development of your eyes and immune system, is another woefully common deficiency in children and pregnant women, with 1 in 6 pregnant women carrying the deficiency, and subsequently 1 in 3 school-age children with it as well.[56] Vitamin A supplementation has, understandably, been found to improve important health biomarkers in deficient children ages 6 - 59 months old as the deficiencies are overcome.[57]

I could go on and on about these types of examples of other common early-life deficiencies in humans like zinc,[58] folate and other B vitamins,[59] as well as the electrolytes like sodium,[60] magnesium,[61] calcium,[62] and potassium,[63] and other trace minerals like selenium[64] but I think you can get the picture.

From birth, most of us are already at a disadvantage.

And it only gets worse from there, with not only the magnitude of these prenatal deficiencies increasing with age, but also the breadth of different deficiencies increasing as well. Meanwhile, as a population we continue to feed our kids nutrient-void foods, and foods rich in anti-nutrients thinking they are healthy, when in fact, they are leeching more and more of these precious micronutrients from our youth.

Malnutrition and micronutrients are major contributors to the global burden of disease,[65] especially in children and mothers.

This undernutrition has been determined to be a major cause of death and disability in young children. "When ranked among other causes, growth faltering and micronutrient deficiencies figure prominently. solid evidence shows that nutrition programs can be effective at addressing nutritional problems in young children."[66]

According to research published in the British Journal of Nutrition, "there is a need for additional measures to increase the intake of certain micronutrients" in children,[67] referencing specifically iron, Vitamin A, and iodine along with zinc, folate and the other B vitamins, as well as the trace mineral selenium.

Micronutrients of all varieties, but especially the prevalent childhood deficiencies such as iodine and selenium, play a central role in the maintenance of metabolism and proper tissue function,[68] so it should come as no surprise that the incidences of metabolic syndrome and epidemic level health issues such as hypothyroidism continue to rapidly rise every decade,[69] with an estimated 20 million Americans having some kind of thyroid disease and over 60% of those individuals not even knowing about their condition.[70] Women, specifically, are up to 8 times more likely to develop a thyroid condition than men, and 1 in 8 women globally are predicted to develop some kind of thyroid condition in their lifetime.[71]

These statistics are alarming!

But we can fix this if we're armed with the right knowledge. But don't go rushing to some popular fad diet either... as they've been found to be one of the leading culprits of micronutrient deficiencies in adult populations.[72]

I will lay out all the proper steps for you to take within the pages of this book, so rest assured - you're in good hands. You've found the right resource.

One of the biggest things you need to be aware of is the presence of something known as anti-nutrients in your current diet. These anti-nutrients quite literally pull crucial micronutrients out of your body - and the worst part is... they're hiding in your "health foods."

Antinutrients

On one hand, as we've discussed, many of us are at a big disadvantage when it comes to nutrient deficiencies either at birth, or by the time we are 6 months old. This is a mixture of a genetic and epigenetic predisposition that we truly can do nothing to control ourselves... it's the "hand we're dealt" so to speak.

We can definitely improve these prenatal deficiencies by influencing people in our own life, namely the education of mothers and soon-to-be mothers, in our friends and family circles.

In terms of immediate impact in your life, this will make the biggest one. The network effect will take care of the rest; the more people who are aware of this issue, the more lives we can impact for the better.

But these early-life deficiencies are not the only cause of micronutrient deficiencies in humans. There are many things that we introduce into our daily habits, specifically foods that we eat, that contain compounds that increase the chances of a nutrient deficiency.

In the case of food, the most powerful *blocker* causing nutrient deficiencies that you're consuming on a daily basis is something known as an antinutrient.

In its strictest sense, antinutrients are compounds found in plants specifically, that either impair your ability to absorb nutrients from that plant, or actually bind to, and pass out crucial nutrients from your own body.[73]

Both of these things can be easily avoided by simply not consuming the foods containing powerful antinutrients.

While many people use the term *antinutrient* loosely to encompass a group of different compounds, there is definitely a spectrum of the magnitude of the effect that these antinutrients can have on the human body.

One antinutrient in particular, has been ranked by researchers as being the #1 most detrimental anti-nutrient to consume for human health, and has been specifically referred to as "possibly the single biggest cause for mineral deficiencies in humans around the world."[74]

This antinutrient is known as phytic acid.

Because of the way phytic acid is chemically-structured, it has a high concentration of negatively charged phosphate groups, which means that when you consume it from certain foods, these negatively charged phosphate groups can easily bind to certain mineral ions which makes them completely unavailable for absorption into your intestines.[74]

With phytic acid, zinc, calcium, and iron are most affected - as found in the research.[75, 76]

The most important step in proper mineral absorption is for the mineral itself to remain in ionic form.[77] When it is bound by an anti-nutrient like phytic acid, it is no longer ionic and therefore can no longer be absorbed by your body.[78]

Phytic acid is well-cited in the scientific literature as a cause for deficiencies with zinc, calcium, and iron,[79-95] and often also for magnesium and copper, however those claims tend to be more controversial.[96]

PHYTIC ACID

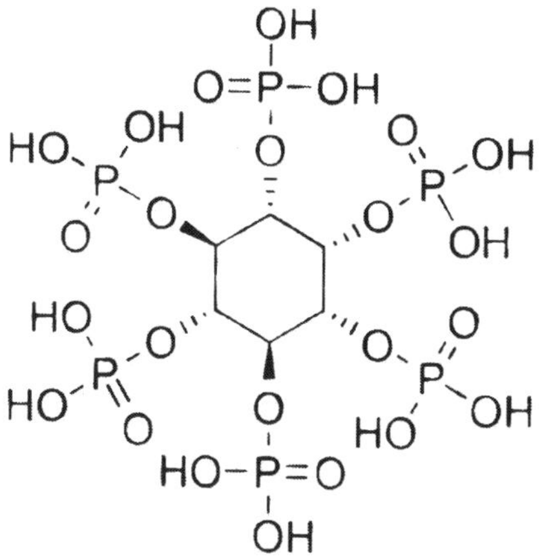

I'll be discussing some important cellular biology in the next chapter with relation to minerals and the key impact they have on our health, so it is also good to note that phytic acid has been shown in research to cause disruption of cell membranes and degradation of DNA,[97] as well as cause pores in the cell membrane itself.

Phytic acid consumption has also been shown to increase the excretion of not just minerals, but also key amino acids, sulphur, nitrogen, and sialic acid.[98] It's also been proven to bind to certain important proteins in the body at specific pH levels.[99]

Because phytic acid is found mostly in plants, and in very high levels in foods like legumes, nuts, seeds and in the bran of grains,[100] researchers have also determined that vegans and vegetarians are at a particularly high risk for nutrient deficiencies,[101] since they tend to rely so heavily on these food sources in their daily dietary intake.

Phytic acid isn't only a culprit in mineral and amino acid excretion, unfortunately. It has also been found to be a potent inhibitor of important bodily enzymes such as trypsin,[102] a proteolytic enzyme that plays an important role in your digestive system.

Phytic acid has also been shown to negatively impact your amylase alpha digestive enzyme,[103, 104] as well as pepsin[105] – the chief digestive enzyme of the stomach.

On top of that, it's been shown to hurt your stomach's ability to digest simple starches.[106]

All-in-all, eating foods high in phytic acid is not recommended for anyone who wants to maintain micronutrient balance and have a healthy digestive system.

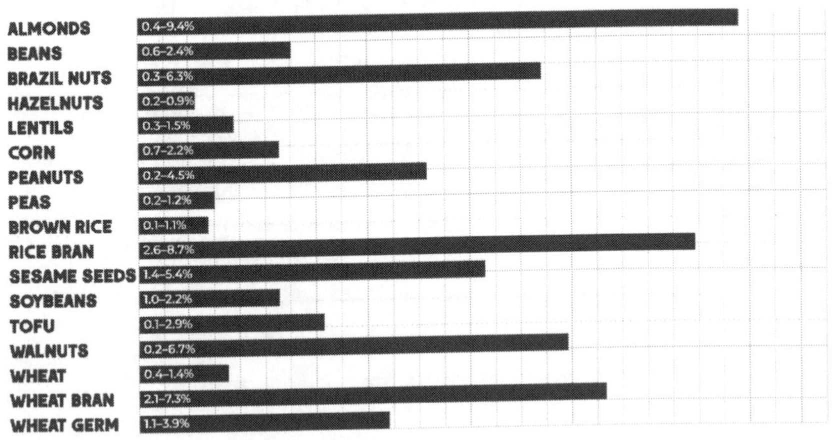

I realize it's controversial to prescribe that you shouldn't eat nuts, beans, whole grains, and seeds, however - according to the scientific research - these foods are leaching important minerals from your body. And not only that, but despite the fact that every me-too health "expert" on the internet tells you they're nutritious - they're actually not. Your body literally cannot access most of the vitamins and minerals inside these foods due to the high anti-nutrient content.

With seeds, for example, researchers have found despite the seed itself containing a lot of different nutrients, the human body can only access magnesium from the seed.[107] All the other nutrients are wasted on us... we cannot digest them. And the phytic acid in the seed can potentially leach minerals from you, so it could be a net negative effect overall. Eating seeds is worse than just wasting your money... they're anti-nutritious.

This isn't even taking the other negative aspects of seeds and nuts into account, such as the extremely high PUFA content, which I discuss in detail in Chapter 4, and the hormone disrupting properties which I discuss in Chapter 7.

Beans are also controversial from the respect that any time I've mentioned legumes being unhealthy on my YouTube channel, a fair amount of angry commenters don't want to hear the truth, but legumes contain not only high amounts of antinutrients, but also high amounts of estrogenic and goitrogenic compounds.[108, 109]

Anything that can reliably damage your thyroid and your reproductive health should be avoided if you agree with me in defining "health" as the ability for your body to be hormonally balanced and to not have any micronutrient deficiencies.

Common Deficiencies That Cause Fat Gain, Lower Your Metabolism, And Hurt Your Ability To Properly Use Sugars

There are a handful of specific deficiencies that negatively affect your metabolism, and have been implicated in complications with metabolic disorders, diabetes, and obesity as well as cause devastating issues with the thyroid gland, which is the master gland for regulating your metabolism.

Magnesium, being one of the most important minerals in your body, understandably plays a major role in your metabolism, along with over 300 other important functions[110] and enzyme systems, including protein synthesis, muscle and nerve function, blood sugar control, and blood pressure regulation.[111, 112]

Magnesium is required for energy production,[113] oxidative phosphorylation,[114] and glycolysis.[115] So it should come as no surprise that a magnesium deficiency would negatively affect all of these important processes in the body, while also causing major downstream negative effects in other systems that need to compensate for the disruption of balance within these systems.

Researchers have also determined that not only is magnesium

deficiency a major role player in the rise of obesity, Type 2 diabetes, metabolic syndrome, osteoporosis, and other inflammation-related disorders, but they also highlight the role of a rising calcium:magnesium ratio.[116] High calcium with low magnesium has been known to be indicative of sympathetic dominance in the body, which is when a person is over-utilizing their sympathetic nervous system; it is a common state of stress fueled by excess adrenaline production[117] that can lead to increased insulin resistance over time.

Vitamin D deficiency is another major player in metabolism and thyroid issues.

One interesting study[118] found that Vitamin D supplementation greatly helped the subjects with glucose metabolism, even in non-obese people, and they determined that this assistance in metabolism was independent of weight or fat mass on the body. This finding highlights the direct impact that Vitamin D has on the metabolic process. Another study in post menopausal women found a similarly important assistance in glucose metabolism with 12 weeks of Vitamin D supplementation.[119]

Vitamin D deficiency is considered a major risk factor for obesity.[120] The prevalence of Vitamin D deficiency in obese individuals ranges[121] between 80-90%.[122] A staggering number - and eye-opening to say the least.

Luckily, researchers are starting to pay attention, and a mounting number of studies are being released to support the fact that Vitamin D deficiency plays a major role in obesity,[123] and correcting this deficiency can help patients to improve their glucose metabolism naturally.

D3 deficiency has been proven to cause pancreatic-β cell dysfunction.[124 - 126]

And numerous studies continue to reinforce the idea of an inverse relationship between Vitamin D levels and the prevalence of Type 2 diabetes in humans.[127 - 132]

Another interesting observation to note is that several researchers have also found that seasonal fluctuations in Vitamin D levels, when in the winter months natural Vitamin D production in the body tends to decline due to less sunlight exposure on the skin, also appears to correlate with seasonal fluctuations in glycemic control in Type 2 diabetics.[133, 134]

So make sure to get plenty of sunlight when you can. And when you cannot, maybe you live in a dismal cold weather climate during the winter months, be sure to consistently supplement with a high quality D3 supplement, preferably suspended in a non-PUFA oil.

Vitamin D3 supplementation has a convincing amount of research to support its use in reversing obesity-related disorders, or aiding in prevention of excessive weight gain in the first place.[135 - 137]

Randomized trials have demonstrated the significant improvements in insulin sensitivity with vitamin D supplementation in patients with insulin resistance or impaired fasting glucose.[138 - 142]

Based on all of this information and clinical support for Vitamin D supplementation in aiding the reversal of insulin resistance, you may want to consider measuring and correcting your Vitamin D deficiencies if you are dealing with this issue.

As far back as the 1950s,[143] chromium was recognized as an essential trace mineral in the insulin signal cascade.[144]

Because of that, unsurprisingly, chromium deficiency has been identified as a common trait in people experiencing issues with severe insulin resistance, high blood sugar, high triglycerides, and neuropathy.[145] Also unsurprisingly, or maybe not so unsurprisingly, research studies have shown a complete and rapid remission of these symptoms when patients supplemented with chromium in high enough quantities and consistently enough to correct their chromium deficiency.[146 - 148]

The human body stores chromium intracellularly in the liver, so liver health is also paramount to protect against a chromium deficiency. The top sources of chromium in foods are in yeast and meat. People with Type 2 diabetes have been found to have between 20-40% lower blood chromium levels[149, 150] and 40-50% lower chromium levels in scalp head and nails[151] compared to healthy people.

When it comes to supplementation, bioavailability always matters, since the body can more readily absorb the nutrient. In the case of chromium, chromium picolinate has been shown to be the only form (and most bioavailable) to consistently demonstrate significant improvements in blood sugar control in clinical trials (13 out of 15 trials).[152] The FDA also approved a health claim for chromium picolinate saying that "it may reduce the risk of insulin resistance."[153]

Thiamine (Vitamin B1)[154] deficiency is another important micronutrient deficiency to pay attention to. This is because it has been found to play a crucial cofactor role in glucose and amino acid metabolism,[155] especially with the three important regulatory enzymes α-keto acid decarboxylase, pyruvate dehydrogenase, and α-ketoglutarate dehydrogenase. These three enzymes regulate the pentose phosphate shunt, glycolysis, and citric acid pathways, respectively.

A thiamine deficiency leads to a reduction in these important pathways, and an increase in certain byproducts that have been shown worsen Type 2 diabetes symptoms and cause endothelial disruption.[156]

When it comes to sources of thiamine, some good food sources are pork, red meat, eggs, and fish.[157] One super interesting thing to note - and this makes perfect sense in the context of what we now know about thiamine's important role in glucose metabolism and its impact on diabetes symptoms - is that when you consume an excessive amount of refined foods, the body uses more thiamine to process it.[158] This becomes troublesome in people who overeat processed foods since these foods also do not contain any thiamine in their chemical makeup. What has become known as the Standard American Diet is woefully void of thiamine and high in processed low-nutrient foods, a ripe formula for disaster, and no-doubt a contributing factor to the steady rise of Type 2 diabetes in the population.

On a diet lacking adequate thiamine, a deficiency can occur in as little as 2-3 weeks with a complete depletion of thiamine from the system[159] - which demonstrates not only how much thiamine is relied upon for your metabolism, but also how dangerous it is to consume a low thiamine diet.

Researchers have done a handful of interesting studies on thiamine deficiency in cultured endothelial cells, demonstrating that in the presence of thiamine, the cells actually lowered their production of ROS[160] (reactive oxygen species, a sign of inflammation) and improved their overall function in a high-glucose environment.[161]

All of this evidence points to the importance of making sure you take measures, whether through diet changes or through supplementation, to ensure you are not deficient in thiamine in order to keep your metabolism operating properly and protect against, or improve, symptoms of Type 2 diabetes.

When it comes to your metabolism, we cannot ignore the role of the thyroid gland.

Your thyroid gland not only regulates your metabolism but is also integrated into other important endocrine feedback loops that affect everything from sexual health to adrenal control over stress hormones to brain health. The American Thyroid Association says that the thyroid "produces a hormone that influences every cell, tissue, and organ in the body."[162] As you can imagine, any nutrient deficiency that negatively impacts your thyroid health can have devastating consequences in other areas of your body as well. The NIH reports that around 5 in every 100 people over the age of 12 in the US has hypothyroidism.[163]

Researchers have found that insufficient supply of thyroid hormones to the developing brain in a fetus can result in mental retardation.[164] In this case, as is true in most cases of thyroid disorder, iodine deficiency plays a major role. Iodine deficiency has the ability to cause brain damage and mental retardation along with a host of other issues in humans.

Your body does not make iodine, so it must be supplied through your diet.[165]

When someone's diet does not supply enough iodine for the body's requirements, a deficiency develops. The thyroid can no longer produce enough thyroid hormone, and therefore sends negative feedback into important endocrine feedback loops, causing a whole host of downstream negative effects.[166]

Iodine interacts with other micronutrients in support of your thyroid gland, specifically Vitamin A,[167] iron,[168] selenium,[168] and zinc.[169] Deficiencies in those micronutrients will therefore also negatively impact your thyroid function.[170]

Micronutrient deficiencies can impact all areas of your life. These deficiencies don't operate in a vacuum; when your brain doesn't work as well as it should, for example - you suffer in all areas of your life. When you're not sexually healthy, this affects you both physically and psychologically. When your thyroid isn't working properly, you gain weight easily, lose your hair, and your well-being is low.

Oftentimes, certain deficiencies can be deduced through observing negative symptoms. This is not the most accurate way to fix your deficiencies but with some trial-and-error, you can definitely get good results. However, if you want to be as accurate as possible, I recommend actually testing for your nutrient deficiencies. A blood or hair analysis will show you the exact micronutrient levels in your body at the time of the test, and you can therefore know the exact target to shoot for in correcting the deficiencies.

Over time of testing regularly, you can also start to see patterns, which can inform better decisions with your nutrition and supplementation regimen. You will notice that when you fix your deficiencies, you start to experience huge improvements in your quality of life rather quickly.

How To Fix Your Nutrient Deficiencies

Luckily, the most difficult part of the battle of overcoming micronutrient deficiencies is actually just overcoming the ignorance around the subject. Once you're aware of the information that I've just demonstrated in this chapter, and once you measure or diagnose your own nutrient deficiencies, it's rather simple and methodical to correct the deficiency through proper dietary modifications and smart supplementation.

I recommend a two step approach to fixing micronutrient deficiencies:

1. Analyze your current diet, and make necessary modifications to support the nutrients you need. For example, if you're currently consuming a lot of anti-nutrient rich foods, take those foods out of your diet. If you realize that you're deficient in magnesium, start to add easily digestible foods into your weekly nutrition plan that include more magnesium. It's a simple thing, but it's essential to modify your diet before moving on to Step 2 since there is a big chance that you're actively consuming *blockers* that are leaching important minerals from your body, or exposing yourself to things or foods on a daily basis that are only moving you in the wrong direction. Get rid of these blockers, and support your new nutrition plan with *activators* that will bring you closer to your state of optimal health by correcting the deficiencies in your diet.

2. Supplement intelligently. What does this mean? Start to view supplementation as a specific science, not so much as a shotgun approach to nutrition. A lot of people just buy supplements as a sort of unmeasured insurance policy. However, a lot of supplements on the market are sold by people who don't know anything about supplements, and also don't care whether the supplements they're selling actually work for you. They just want to make money. On the other hand, there are certain brands that truly do care about the quality of their products - these brands are much more rare and special. They care about the bioavailability of their nutrients, the synergy and design of their formulas, and they care a lot about improving the health of their customers. You just need to find those brands. My company UMZU is one of those. Our mission is entirely based around helping our customers with the best products possible, along with investing a lot of time, energy, and resources into educating our customers so you can make the best decisions possible for yourself. Smart supplementation entails finding the most bioavailable forms of the nutrients you need, and supplementing with them in the correct dosages in order to fix your deficiency quickly and safely.

To help you find the best foods and supplements possible to correct your micronutrient deficiencies, and arm you with the knowledge and nutrition habits so you never have to deal with these pesky deficiencies again, I put together a detailed table for you highlighting every major micronutrient deficiency you could possibly have, along with the best foods for you to eat to correct this specific deficiency as well as the most bioavailable forms of these nutrients that you should use.

CHAPTER TWO

EAT MORE SALT

THE LAW OF ELECTROCHEMICAL SIGNALING

Misinformation has spread the lie that salt is bad for people. Nothing could be further from the truth. Salt is key to life. When most people hear the word 'salt' they immediately imagine table salt, or sodium chloride. Sodium is not the only salt-forming mineral, however. Electrolytes such as magnesium, potassium, and calcium also form salts. As discussed in Chapter 1, deficiencies in the electrolytes can have devastating effects on the human body. Limiting salt in your diet increases the risk of hyponatremia, mineral deficiencies, hypertension, poor neuronal functioning, fat storage, heart attack, and poor sleep. Most of us don't need to eat a low-salt diet; in fact, we need MORE salt in our diets to improve our health. Stop ignoring your salt cravings while you opt for "low sodium" tasteless foods and bland meals - allow your salt cravings to guide you toward a state of perfect health. Your body is speaking to you - it is time to start listening.

By the turn of the century, the "low salt" diet myth had been thoroughly disproven in the medical literature,[1] drawing upon evidence from hundreds of contradictory studies and reviews, however the myth pervades conventional medical advice and media attention to this day.[2]

Even the US federal and state governments via the FDA and US Department of Health and Human Services, with a seemingly endless stream of high profile initiatives led by power hungry politicians and regulators, have been openly advocating for the general public to lower their salt consumption.[3]

For example, by 2010, Michael Bloomberg, mayor of New York City, convinced 16 food companies to lower the salt levels in their food manufacturing[4] and medical associations like the Institute of Medicine were lobbying the FDA for nation-wide regulations.[5]

But why?

Where did this theory come from? Do we really need to eat less salt to be healthier and why is the government involved?

Like all great conventional health wisdom of the last hundreds years, the salt myth finds its origins in the development and distribution of pharmaceutical drugs.

It all started with syphilis...[6]

From as long ago as the 16th century, mercury had been used throughout Europe for the treatment of syphilis,[7] the sexually transmitted bacterial infection that rose to epidemic levels after Christopher Colombus' second homecoming to Spain in 1497.[8] Mercury is rapidly absorbed in the bodily areas commonly affected by syphilis - the rectum,[9] genitals,[10] and mouth[11] - and was used for hundreds of years to kill the bacteria.

As you can imagine, mercury treatments are not exactly safe, leading to a host of other heavy metal toxicity symptoms, including sudden death[12] (with no warning indicators) and rapid onset of severe diseases including nephrotic syndrome,[13] or kidney failure. However, use of this treatment spread across Europe and was widely used up until the 1950s, when the US pharmaceutical industry made headway with safer alternative drug development and stopped using mercury and arsenic as antibiotics, replacing them with penicillin[14] which was discovered by Alexander Fleming in 1928.[15]

One key element to note about the mercury treatments was that they were diuretics - officially known as *mercurial diuretics.*

With the development of new diuretic treatments, beyond common historically used organic xanthine diuretics such as caffeine, theobromine, and theophylline which can be easily extracted from plant sources,[16] drug companies began to notice other applications.

The first modern diuretic drug of the 1950s, acetazolamide,[17] a carbonic anhydrase inhibitor, proved an exciting entry into the subsequent development of chlorothiazide,[18] furosemide,[19] and ethacrynic acid.[20]

Scientists soon realized that these drugs had the ability to be prescribed widely for use in many clinical applications, including treatments for hypertension,[21] heart failure,[22] many forms of edema,[23] and even obesity.[24]

They also began prescribing these diuretic drugs to pregnant women with the purpose of decreasing water retention during pregnancy.[25]

At the same time, Walter Kempner, a Duke University scientist who had fled Nazi Germany during WWII, began developing and testing a novel dietary protocol for decreasing blood pressure, with a strict focus on white rice and fruit intake.[26] The lack of salt consumption in his diet protocol quickly led to discussions in the medical literature about salt's role in hypertension, and the popular sentiment quickly led to physicians accompanying their prescriptions of the aforementioned diuretic drugs alongside a recommendation that the patients also eat a "low salt diet" for maximum effectiveness of the diuretic effect, since diuretics chiefly act to excrete sodium in the urine.

Salt restriction, however, is extremely damaging to the prenatal development of the fetus in the womb,[27] and it became well-known by more discerning scientists and physicians that these recommendations, especially to pregnant women, would lead to widespread damage to millions of newborn children.

By reducing salt intake during pregnancy, the developing fetus is not receiving adequate oxygen, due to the lowered blood volume, since sodium is essential for maintaining blood volume. The low sodium in the body also prevents enough blood from circulating through the kidneys,[28] which causes the kidneys to release more renin, a signaling enzyme, which is a compensation mechanism the body uses to increase blood pressure in order to circulate blood more quickly.

This lack of oxygen to the growing fetus, and the resulting reduction in CO2 production, not surprisingly, can lead to developmental disorders in the child and postpartum hormonal imbalances in the mother, which commonly symptomize in the forms of hair loss, depression, and skin issues.[29]

The opposition to mass prescription of modern diuretics and low salt diets was mounting, however diuretic drug sales continued to prove massively profitable for the drug companies, and the low salt diet myth quickly became the conventional cliche, parroted in the popular media and throughout doctors' offices around the country.

The ball was already rolling down the hill, and with so much profit to fuel its acceleration, it became impossible to stop.

But is salt really the cause of hypertension or edema?

In short, no. The castle was built on a foundation of sand.

While it's easy to find an array of studies demonstrating small drops in blood pressure with lowered salt intake, these results do not necessarily indicate any sort of causative role of salt consumption in high blood pressure. The results seen are typically so minimal that it becomes obvious to a scrupulous eye that there is a more intricate story at play.

For example, the Department of Health and Human Services funded an 11 trial salt restriction study executed by the Cochrane Collaboration in 2004,[30] that demonstrated an average of just a 1.1 mmHg drop in systolic blood pressure and 0.6 mmHg drop in diastolic blood pressure with salt restriction in healthy humans. This is basically going from 120/80 to 118.9/79.4, results that can easily be achieved in any number of ways.

However, the headlines in popular media outlets chimed out the bells that *"Salt causes high blood pressure!"* further perpetuating the myth in the public's mind and within the medical community, while continuing to ignore highly contradictory results from other wide scale population studies, such as the Intersalt Study of 1988,[31] a data-driven collection of results from 52 international research centers, that demonstrated that the highest salt-consuming individuals (up to 14g of salt per day) *had lower blood pressure levels on average* than people who consumed half of that amount.

The results of the 2004 government-funded Cochrane study,

and ensuing media attention, become even more tenuous when you understand that the Cochrane Collaboration had conducted a study just one year prior, in 2003, reviewing 57 salt restriction trials, and concluded that *"there is little evidence for long-term benefit from reducing salt intake."*[32]

A large study done in 1995 on 3000 people over 4 years led by Dr. Michael Alderman, and published in the journal *Hypertension*,[33] demonstrated that individuals who ate less salt indeed actually had a *higher prevalence of increased mortality rates* than those who ate more salt. They also found that by adding more salt to their diet, the subjects had a 36% decrease in heart-related mortality events.

Three years later, in 1998, the Alderman team published another set of findings on a 22 year long study they'd been conducting with over 11,000 people that showed *a clear inverse relationship* between salt intake and mortality.[34]

In basic biochemistry, it's well-understood that the breakdown of ATP to ADP + phosphate is required for the cell to use glucose and oxygen in order to maintain homeostatic functioning of the body's core metabolic processes.[35]

This breakdown to ADP and phosphate cannot happen without the presence of adequate sodium in the fluid around the cell.[36]

The more sodium present in this fluid, the better the cell is able to increase its energy consumption, which leads to more CO2 production, fueling the metabolism properly and balancing the effects of intracellular calcium.

When unchecked by sodium, and the resulting lack of CO_2 production, calcium can exert toxic effects on the cell,[37] causing premature cell death. All of these compounds must be present in healthy levels in order to ensure the proper functioning and movement of ions through ion channels on the membrane.

Put simply, you need sodium. Badly.

At this point, I think it might be helpful to take a moment and *clearly define what salt actually is,* in order to better enrich your understanding of how important it is to your health.

Think back to high school chemistry class, when you learned about ions. You may recall discussions about anions and cations, usually paired with anxiety-inducing equations on your final exams.

Cations (cat-eye-ons) are ions with a **net positive charge.**[38] They have more protons (positive charge) than electrons (negative charge).

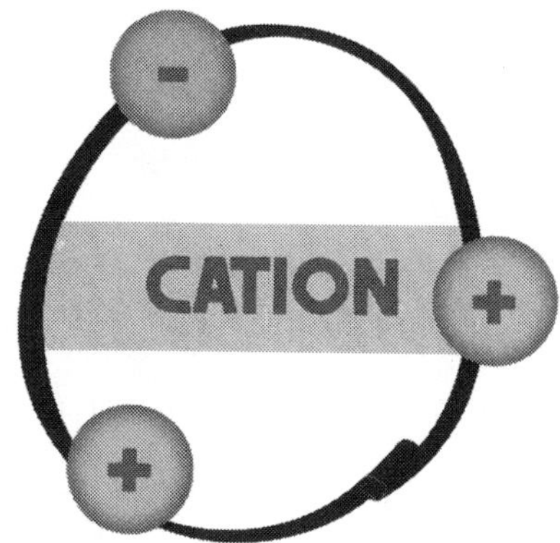

Anions (an-eye-ons) are simply ions with a **net negative overall charge**.[39] They have more electrons (negative charge) than protons (positive charge).

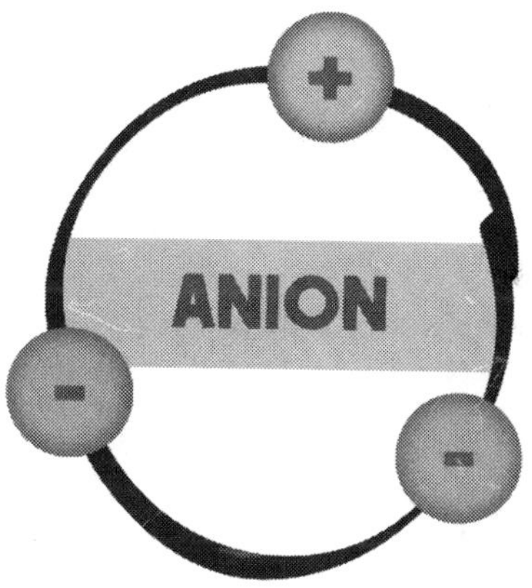

Easy, right?

An *ion* itself is really just an atom or molecule that carries an electrical charge.[40]

Our bodies are like big, organic magnets. The principles of

electromagnetism apply to us, just like they apply to the U-shaped polar magnets we used to play with as children to grab metal paper clips off the ground.

Every second of every day, millions of imperceptible ionic reactions are taking place inside you. They're vitally important to your survival. If they all stopped happening, even just for a second, you would die on the spot.

A *salt*, then, is quite simply the chemical compound that is created when a cation and anion are attracted to one another due to opposing charges and join together in a chemical reaction in order to reach a net neutral charge.[41]

Let's take table salt for example... NaCL.

The cation, sodium (Na+) carries a net +1 positive charge. The chloride (Cl-) carries a net -1 negative charge. Combine them together and boom, you have table salt with a net neutral charge.

Since naming conventions indicate that the cation must be first and the anion second,[42] it's common for people to refer to salts simply by using the cation, like "sodium." However, it's important to know that there can be many different types of sodium-based salts, and the same is true with other cations such as calcium, magnesium, and potassium.

Salt itself is so essential to the human body, that "saltiness" is one of the 5 classifications of perceptible taste by taste receptors on the tongue,[43] and so essential to life in general, that it is the main mineral constituent of ocean water and a huge part of the Earth's crust, especially underwater, where hydrothermal vents in the oceanic crust, basalt, continually pump minerals into the ocean from the Earth's surface.[44]

Restricting your salt intake compromises your body's ability to function properly, especially on the cellular level.

Any sort of dysfunction at this micro level can have wide-reaching negative effects on the macro level as the body's natural compensation mechanisms kick in to attempt to overcome the lack of salt it requires. For example, I previously mentioned that when the kidneys don't have enough blood flow, which is facilitated by sodium, they will compensate by releasing a signaling enzyme called renin to increase blood pressure in an attempt to bring more blood to the kidneys.

This leads to a full activation of the RAAS, or the renin-angiotensin-aldosterone system, which quickly increases risk of hypertension,[45] kidney problems,[46] heart complications,[47] and rapidly increases serotonin production,[48] another poorly-understood, insidious health issue I will discuss in more detail later in this book.

Long story short, salt restriction actually *causes* the very health issues the medical community believes it solves. This is just one of many examples highlighting the dangers of parroting conventional wisdom cliches, a multi-generation propagation of misinformation that continues to harm millions of people's lives.

When your body has enough salt, you reap the rewards of vibrant health. You move closer to the *Thermo State* effortlessly. Your body is a self-healing organism; provide it with the raw materials it needs to operate correctly.

The next time you reach for that extra pinch of salt to enhance your food's taste, think of it as a daily ritual to support a faster metabolism, lower stress hormone levels, and lower inflammation.

That extra pinch of salt can also protect your brain against anxiety and depression while improving your brain's ability to learn new things and retain information.

By following the simple nutrition tenets outlined within these pages, your body will efficiently use glucose as a metabolic fuel, supporting healthy functioning of important organs like your thyroid, pituitary, kidneys, heart, and liver.

When your body is using glucose properly, your metabolic rate increases rapidly,[49] and the self-healing properties kick-in, which brings your health back into balance. When your body is not using glucose properly, free fatty-acids start dumping into the blood as an alternate fuel source,[50] which requires a systemic increase in stress hormones cortisol, estrogen, and adrenaline, which serve to catabolize tissue and slow down your metabolism while compromising the basic functioning of those vital organs.

Because of this reality, the fatty-acid metabolism is also known as the "survival state," where reproductive function decreases, metabolic rate decreases, blood pressure increases, blood sugar issues become dysfunctional, and vital organ functioning slows down... all in your body's interest of preserving resources.

In 2011, a detailed meta-analysis of 6250 human subjects published in the American Journal of Hypertension found no evidence to conclude that salt restriction helped people lower their risk of high blood pressure, heart attacks, or stroke.[51]

A few months prior to those findings, another study published in the Journal of the American Medical Association concluded that lower salt intake increases the risk of premature death from heart complications.[52]

The interesting thing to note here, is that those medical journals are well-known and respected resources in both the US and international medical communities, and receive government funding, however their findings on analysis of the salt restriction myth continue to fall on deaf ears within those same communities because of the deeply-entrenched groupthink that has been established for so many decades to this point.

In 2006, the Journal of American Medicine published their findings on a massive analysis of the salt consumption of 78 million Americans over 14 years, reporting that, much to the chagrin of the proponents of the conventional wisdom on the subject, *the more sodium a person ate, the lower their risk of dying from heart disease.*[53]

By consuming salt regularly, your cells function properly, utilizing glucose for fuel and shuttling more oxygen through the blood to your vital organs. Blood pressure normalizes and the thyroid gland is able to produce plenty of thyroid hormone T4 to maintain a well-regulated metabolic feedback loop.[54]

Sodium has a thermogenic effect within the body. By increasing overall body temperature, it increases the metabolic rate of brown fat by increasing the activity of the fat synthesizing enzyme.[55] This sodium-induced increase in metabolization of brown fat also interestingly improves sleep, since it improves production of the inhibitory neurotransmitter GABA,[56] which gives you a nice sedative effect when you're ready to relax and lay down for a good night's sleep.

An increase in brown fat metabolism has been shown to improve slow wave sleep (SWS),[57] known colloquially as *deep sleep,* which is the deepest form of NREM sleep, where most of the body's recovery mechanisms kick-in, such as pulsatile release of growth hormone, and when learning and memory consolidation happens. During SWS, all of the neuronal connections that were made during the waking hours of the day via long-term potentiation, are given a chance to consolidate, and the brain is able to prune the weakly-potentiated synaptic connections, strengthening the more useful connections. SWS is vital for this learning and memory process, *synaptic plasticity.*[58]

How much salt should you eat?

Remember, you need to regularly consume the right amount of salt in order to allow the sodium to regulate calcium in the cell and prevent excess electrolyte loss in general.

The average person will need to consume roughly 60–65mg/kg body weight of salt daily in order to maintain the proper balance of sodium to calcium, magnesium, and potassium in the cellular milieu.

Salt is roughly 40% sodium, so the typical person, depending on body weight, needs 10–15g per day in their diet. If you're consuming baking soda, sodium bicarbonate, you will need 20–22g daily, since it is roughly 27% sodium.

Yes, these recommendations are well above the government RDA guidelines. And that's the whole point. Government guidelines are wrong.

These recommendations are especially important if you're an athlete and/or you exercise regularly, since studies have shown that athletes can lose up to 30g of sodium per day,[59] which will clearly impair your physical performance since these levels of sodium loss can wreak havoc on fluid balance and your body's ability to use glucose properly.

Dropping below 3-5g of salt intake per day, depending on body weight, has been shown to actually *increase water retention*, due to the decrease in overall blood volume and oxygen delivery.[60]

The bottom line... Eat more salt.

Stop restricting your salt intake. Sodium is necessary for your body to function properly, starting at the most basic cellular level. Adequate sodium in your diet allows your cells to use fuel properly, releasing energy and oxygen, so you can subsequently produce more carbon dioxide which brings order to your tissues, organs, and ultimately your entire organism. By increasing your daily salt intake, not only will your meals taste more delicious, but you will actively support a healthy thyroid gland, a higher body temperature, a faster metabolism, more brown fat burning, better sleep, normal blood pressure, and a fertile reproductive system.

Salt is your friend.

CHAPTER THREE

EAT SUGAR

THE LAW OF METABOLIC PREFERENCE

Sugar is not bad; it is essential to health. The cell needs glucose in order to function properly in an anti-stress state with high energy flow. Research supports the idea that carbohydrates are needed to "thrive". The modern demonization of sugar is entirely based on a complete and utter misunderstanding of what sugar is, and its vital roles in the human body. Half of the problem in understanding (anything) is based in language - definitions, and a knowledge gap between assumptions and reality. The knowledge gap, characterized by ignorance, is a result of "received wisdom." Enlightenment is born out of critical re-examination of our previously held beliefs, which are almost always beliefs that slither into the deep recesses of our minds without our conscious acceptance or rejection. If enough authorities echo the same sentiment, it must be true... right? The beliefs currently held by the majority of Western society about sugar are all based in received wisdom, and are inaccurate. These inaccurate beliefs pour gasoline on an already epidemic-level fire of chronic health issues in hundreds of millions of people. Myths around cancer, diabetes, insulin reactivity, and ketosis are keeping the wool pulled over the eyes of millions of people who need help! Enhance your understanding of the reality of sugar's role in the human body, and you will unlock the door to optimal thyroid function, insulin sensitivity, mitochondrial efficiency, and low stress hormones. Start using sugar properly, from the right sources, and the resulting body fat loss, boundless energy, high sex hormones, mental clarity, and incredible sleep will completely change your life for the better.

In 1938, the results of a 6-month long study were published in The Journal Of Nutrition[1]... and the lab that published them was at a critical crossroads, one that would set the wheels in motion for the public's understanding - or rather misunderstanding - around human health for the next 80 years.

The results of the study most certainly would've been "disturbing" to the researchers, primarily because they indicated the opposite of what the researchers set out to prove.

Were true scientific methodology the guiding light, these results would have necessitated a different path than the one that was chosen. But there was a lot at stake, and these results were inconvenient. As stated in the Advancement of Learning, *"if a man will begin with certainties, he shall end in doubts; but if he will be content to begin with doubts, he shall end in certainties."*[2]

The lab of George Burr had started with certainties, and ended in doubts. But it wasn't long before those doubts were forgotten, stamped out by the unbridled force of their original certainties.

The mental and biological constructs at work in the brain to ensure what scientists call "certainty bias" are of the strongest kind of misdirected superpower. Robert Burton M.D., former Chief of Neurology at the University of California at San Francisco, points out that "we need to recognize that the feelings of certainty and conviction are involuntary mental sensations, not logical conclusions."[3]

Burton points out[4] that there are two separate aspects of a thought: the actual thought and an independent involuntary assessment of the accuracy of that thought. The brain has powerful built-in involuntary mechanisms for unconscious cognitive activity. Many thoughts that surface in someone's mind, researchers included, are driven from this not-necessarily-logical unconscious inroad... what William James, the Father of American Psychology and professor of philosophy at Harvard University, referred to in his Gifford Lectures as "felt knowledge."[5]

Often this "felt knowledge" is much stronger than a logical conclusion, and will drive human behavior far beyond the rigid regulations of logical thought, even when that person is staring directly into the cold, unblinking eyes of a conflicting truth... potentially to their own demise, or worse, to the demise of others.

It is entirely possible that the Burr laboratory in the 1930's was driven chiefly by "felt knowledge" - in fact, the evolution of their theories birthed at that time would indicate as much, including the fact that they "invented" a disease - the resulting turn of events - part-scientific, part-political, and part-blind-ambition - spawned a divergence from the truth that nobody could have possibly predicted the effects of at that time.

So what happened?

In the early 1930's, years before the publication of the aforementioned study, Burr was running experiments related to his theory of "essential fatty acid deficiency" in rats. He noticed that PUFA-deficient rats on a specific high sugar diet consumed oxygen at an uncharacteristically high rate.[6]

Burr erroneously concluded that first, this increased consumption of oxygen was a bad thing, which was based on a foundational misunderstanding and bias that was brought into the experiment. Secondly, he observed that it was due to a lack of unsaturated fats in the animals' diet. His reasoning was that this lack of unsaturated fats increased the rate at which water escapes as vapor through the skin of the rats, and that, because of this, the so-called "essential fatty acid deficiency" must be overcome in order to slow this rate of evaporation.

His observations missed some key pieces to the puzzle. It was the 1930s afterall, and scientific understanding of the human body has advanced massively since then (in some areas, while devolving in others).

He didn't understand that the amount of water evaporated from an animal's body is actually a reliable indicator of metabolic rate, a direct function of a healthy thyroid gland! The animals were healthier without the "essential fatty acids" in their diet. When an animal's metabolic rate is higher, it burns calories at a higher rate, creating more heat. The body's natural response is to leverage the sweat glands to help the animal maintain a steady body temperature... and evaporation is the main cooling mechanism.

He threw the baby out with the bathwater!

This is where William Brown entered the picture in 1938. Working as a researcher in Burr's lab, Brown became curious about the effects of this "essential fatty acid deficient" diet. What type of impact would it have on humans? To that point, it had only been measured on animals.

He decided to put it to the test on himself.

For 6 months Brown consumed a 2500 calorie per day diet completely void of unsaturated fats, and high in sugars in the forms of glucose, fructose, lactose, sucrose, and potato starch along with micronutrient supplementation from mineral oil, baking soda, and salt, as well as Vitamin D3, Vitamin A, and iron.

Despite the fact that the Burr laboratory was clutching onto the idea that a diet without unsaturated fatty acids was "unhealthy" and caused the fake disease (of their own invention) "essential fatty acid deficiency," the results from Brown's study were undeniable: this diet made him healthier.

First, Brown had suffered since childhood from migraines. Within 6 weeks on this high sugar diet, they completely subsided and never returned. Secondly, he started the diet with slightly high blood pressure. A few months into the experimental diet, his blood pressure completely normalized.

He also lost a significant amount of weight through the 6 month period, corresponding to a measurable increase in his metabolic rate indicators. He went from 152lbs at the start of the dieting period with a metabolic rate at -12% below normal, and within a few months raised his metabolic rate to just -2% below normal while dropping to 138lbs, which he easily maintained through the end of the study period.

At 2500 calories per day, mostly from sugar, this is a feat most people would not believe possible, especially at his body weight and without extra activity.

Brown also reported a noticeable increase in energy throughout his work days. Where he used to feel a sense of fatigue at the end of the day, he reported that this fatigue completely disappeared while on the diet.

And similar to the rats, his respiratory quotient significantly increased, which also indicates an increase in metabolic rate and thyroid function. His respiratory quotient was above a 1.0, hitting as high as 1.14 during the sixth month of the experiment.

A respiratory quotient of 1.0 and above indicates an exceptional ability of the body to oxidize pure carbohydrate for fuel. Juxtapose this against the respiratory quotient of a Type 2 diabetic, which can fall down into the 0.7 range, indicative of a preference in the diabetic physiology of oxidizing fatty acids instead of carbohydrates.

And weirdly, despite their reporting that the diet didn't significantly change Brown's cholesterol measurements, it actually dropped his total serum cholesterol quite a bit, going from 298 to 206 mg/dL over the first four months. That's significant in my book.

Despite these findings of lack of fatty acids, and a higher sugar diet actually improving health biomarkers in both the animals and in Brown's six month human trial, Burr pushed forward and continued to assert his "essential fatty acid deficiency" hypothesis. Funny enough, it mostly fell on deaf ears in the scientific community at the time, since many other researchers were corroborating similar positive health results of the opposite of what Burr was claiming with his fatty acid hypothesis. The other researchers at the time were finding that as the thyroid gland improved functioning through a higher sugar diet and lower polyunsaturated fats, the serum cholesterol numbers also normalized into the healthy range.

Unfortunately, this was all forgotten when the Seed Oil industry stepped into the picture, and changed the course of Western society for the remainder of the century. I discuss this sad historical phenomenon in detail in the chapter on PUFAs, but to sum it up in the context of Burr and his "essential fatty acid deficiency" hypothesis, once cottonseed oil no longer had a distribution in the paint industry, the massive surplus of this oil and other "vegetable oils" in the US in the early 1900s spurred the marketing of it as a food product, with a steady introduction into the American food supply, primarily via companies like Wesson, J.M Smucker, and Procter & Gamble.

The essential fatty acid deficiency hypothesis was the perfect marketing fodder to prop up a "scientific" argument for why Americans should start consuming vegetable oils en masse, since these vegetable oils are entirely made up of the same fatty acids as Burr was asserting to be "essential" - polyunsaturated fats, or PUFAs.

The very fact that they became referred to as "vegetable" oils is also a misnomer and a testament to the propaganda influence behind this early 20th century movement in corporate food marketing, especially since none of these oils are actually taken from vegetables, but rather seeds.

"If you are deficient in these essential vegetable oils, you cannot possibly be healthy," the propaganda began to spread like wildfire, to the tune of billions in profits, no doubt with the help of the prodigal propagandist Edward Bernays,[7] a nephew of Sigmund Freud, who worked with companies like Procter & Gamble during this time, and who is also well-known for the central role he played in convincing the American public that water fluoridation was healthy and necessary (he was hired by the special interest group Alcoa - the Aluminum Company of America to do this), that cigarettes were cool, and in working with the large multinational corporation United Fruit Company (now named Chiquita Brands International) and the US government (the CIA, President Eisenhower, and Secretary of State John Foster Dulles) to overthrow the democratically-elected president of Guatemala, Jacobo Arbenz Guzman - who took a hard line against the United Fruit Companies exploitative labor practices in Guatemala, in operation PBSUCCESS in 1954.

It's important to understand the historical sequence of events here, as well as the players involved, in order to have an accurate basis for your decision making around sugar, especially since sugar, vegetable oils and "essential" fatty acids, cholesterol, and heart disease are all such intricately tied topics when it comes to the propaganda and marketing milieu of the 20th and 21st centuries.

This sequence of events made certain corporations massive amounts of money, setting them up to be in the top most influential and powerful companies on Earth now in the 21st century, while also causing a massive confusion within the medical, scientific, and research communities... trickling down to the general public and no doubt correlating - and I would even go so far as to suggest a causal role - with the epidemic rise of chronic metabolic disease in the world population over the last 100 years, with obesity tripling since 1975, where more than 1 in 3 adults are now overweight, and over 340 million children were found to be overweight in a 2016 population survey.[8]

Why does everyone still believe sugar is bad for the body, especially when sugar consumption is actually decreasing while the rates of obesity and Type 2 diabetes continue to rise?

The idea that eating sugar causes obesity, Type 2 diabetes, and cancer is a pre scientific belief, perpetuated through the last few centuries to the detriment of hundreds of millions of people. The development of this "sugar disease" theory rode alongside, and relied heavily upon, the veracity of the lipid theory of heart disease, which indicts cholesterol and saturated fat consumption as causal factors in cardiovascular disease, and, despite the fact that these theories have both been thoroughly disproven,[9] these inaccurate ideas remain firmly seated on the dogmatic throne at the center of the temple of the cultural hive mind, held as immutable truth.

To paint an accurate picture of reality, we must understand the origin of these debunked theories. Confucius put it simply, *"study the past if you would define the future."*

Everyone loves to demonize sugar as the cause of obesity, yet when you analyze both the research and the actual biochemistry of the human body, you start to see a very different picture unfold, with some extremely convincing evidence to the contrary.

People rarely ever consume sugar in its pure form.

When was the last time you ate a spoonful of raw coconut or maple sugar, or real honey? For many people, probably never.

First off, sugar does not equal baked goods, candy bars, soft drinks, and anything else people commonly associate it with.

It is NOT the same thing.

All of these foodstuffs are nothing more than nutrient-void garbage food that should be consumed sparingly, if at all. They contain large amounts of polyunsaturated fats, grain flours, and frankenfood ingredients and flavoring chemicals that negatively influence your health far more than a little sucrose.

This is the real crime in implicating "sugar" as something that's bad for the body...

Because the baby gets thrown out with the bathwater...

People, by association, demonize fruit, honey, and even just simple raw cane sugar, with zero real evidence for its negative effects in the context of an otherwise solid hormonally-focused diet like I outline in this book.

Rarely do people fully understand what sugar is, how it acts in the body, and how much it really contributes to obesity, inflammation, hormones, etc. And now that we've moved over from blaming saturated fat for all of our health problems, we need a new thing to demonize and blame for our obesity and health problems.

Sugar is the perfect target, and it certainly gets its share of a bad rep already.

But did you know that even though we try to blame sugar for everything, and say that we are getting fatter and fatter due to increased sugar usage, science actually shows that sugar consumption has dropped during this time that obesity rates have dramatically risen.

One study[10] calls this *"the Australian Paradox"*, as during the timeframe of 1980–2003, obesity rates tripled in the country, yet the intake of refined sugar dropped by 23%.

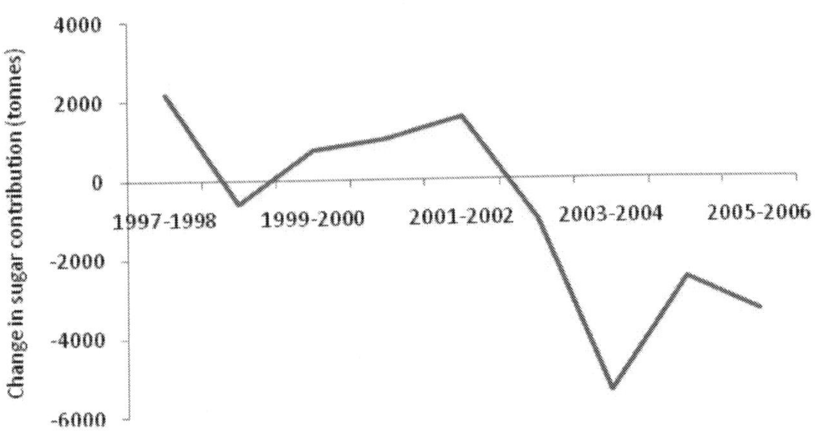

What is Sugar

Sugars are naturally occurring carbohydrates that provide energy for the body in the form of glucose and fructose. Your brain, for example, requires roughly 120 grams of glucose on a daily basis to cover the most basic energy needs.[11]

The major internal organs, glands, and muscles all use glucose as their main energy source. If you deprive the body from this, it will try to make up for it by a process called gluconeogenesis, in which the body breaks down protein and fatty-acids to create glucose. Do this long enough and your body goes into ketosis, which is just another form of metabolic stress during glucose deprivation.

Almost all carbohydrates, starches and sugars, break down to glucose – the simplest form of sugar – after ingestion. The rate at which this happens is measured by the *"glycemic index"* or *"glycemic load"*.

Although the low-carbers tried for years to confuse average people into believing that low glycemic index foods would be "it" for weight loss. Research has shown time after time again that it was the total energy intake of daily calories, not the GI that is behind our ability to gain or lose weight.[12]

The most common kinds of sugars in our diet include:

- **Glucose** – the simplest form of sugar and the main energy provider of the cells in the body. The "blood sugar" in your veins is also glucose.

- **Fructose** – found naturally in fruits and honey. It's much sweeter than glucose and is metabolized in the liver instead of the gut.
- **Sucrose** – (table sugar) is 50% fructose and 50% glucose, extracted from beets or sugar cane. Sucrose occurs naturally in vegetables and fruit.
- **Lactose** – (milk sugar) is found in milk and dairy products. There's also maltose, which is found in malted drinks and beer.

The studies looking into the effects of sugar on various health parameters, often use pure fructose, pure glucose, or sucrose. In our normal daily lives, the majority of the sugars we consume come in balance of ~50% glucose, ~50% fructose. The main difference between glucose and fructose, is the fact that the latter is metabolized in the liver and is more rapidly absorbed.

The best possible way to fully understand sugar, is to understand the structure and function of carbohydrates inside the human body.

Carbohydrates are organic compounds that contain carbon, hydrogen, and oxygen.[13] A convenient shorthand that scientists use to reference a carbohydrate, or carbohydrate-fed subject group, in the literature is CHO (carbon-hydrogen-oxygen).

Carbohydrates are the most abundant biomolecule on Earth and they're used for accessible energy to fuel cellular reactions and for vital structural support of cell membranes. The presence of the carbohydrate enhances the ability of the cell to not just function at baseline, but to be able to improve its functionality over time - as long as it has a steady access to a source of carbohydrate.

For example,[14] a cell can use a carbohydrate molecule to bind to the lipids in the cell membrane to improve cell identification, cell signaling, and cellular immune responses.

Certain forms of carbohydrates such as deoxyribose and ribose are essential parts of DNA and RNA molecules' structure and function.[15]

There are thousands of different carbohydrate forms, but they all consist of one or more units called monosaccharides.

Monosaccharides are named accordingly, with Greek roots, as "simple sugars." The number and type of monosaccharide used - as well as the positioning of how they're bonded with one another - determines the structure of a carbohydrate.

For example, sucrose (table sugar) is known as a disaccharide, and is formed by the bonding of two monosaccharides, glucose and fructose.

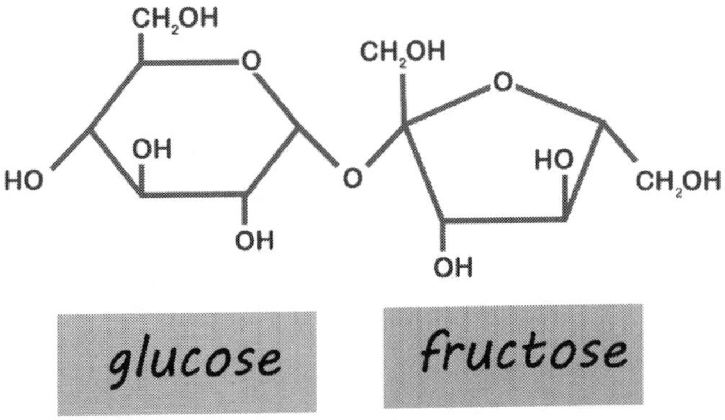

Different monosaccharide pairs form a lot of the common sugars we associate with foods: such as sucrose, maltose (two glucose monomers), and lactose (glucose and galactose monomers).

Polysaccharides - also known as "complex carbohydrates" - consist of chains of hundreds of more monosaccharide units,[16] and they're usually - but not always - composed of the same type of monosaccharides, such as glucose, linked together in different numbers.

Polysaccharides are great for energy use and storage in the human body since they're so easily built and broken down by enzymes naturally found within the body. We create glucose polymers to be stored as energy in the form of glycogen in the liver and muscle tissue. This allows it to be stored in a compact surface area, but provides large amounts of easily available energy when needed. Since glycogen is such a heavily relied upon source of energy in the body, especially in times of urgent need, glycogen depletion - when we don't consume enough glucose in our diet, or when we intentionally run our glycogen stores low - can cause detrimental side effects in energy production, most commonly described as "hitting the wall" or "bonking" in athletics.

When the body is fully depleted of glycogen, a shift in stress hormone production facilitates a process known as gluconeogenesis, or the creation of glucose from lactate, pyruvate, and amino acids,[17] and is characteristic of a catabolic, or stressed, metabolism.

Gluconeogenesis is a survival mechanism ingrained in the body that can help keep the organism alive in the absence of glucose-rich food. It requires a highly stressed and catabolic shift in certain hormone production such as cortisol and adrenaline, and is not preferable for a healthy long-term condition. Many people report "feeling great" for a short period of time after this hormonal shift, however this feeling of well-being is also a survival mechanism for the animal, and is commonly known as the "catecholamine honeymoon",[18] characterized by a sharp rise in catecholamines, like adrenaline, followed by the decreased sensitivity to such hormones, despite their chronically-elevated levels of release into the blood in order to sustain gluconeogenesis in the absence of glucose.

After as short as just a few weeks in this condition, the negative effects of these catabolic stress hormones become quite noticeable - decreases in energy, hair thinning, insomnia, loss of sex drive, loss of muscle tissue, and stubborn body fat. You could say, the honeymoon is over at that point.

Due to the demonization of sugar, it may seem a bit outer-worldish to claim that sugar consumption would actually have some health benefits.

Yet it does. And it makes sense.

There's plenty of research showing how glucose and fructose actually negatively correlate with diabetes,[19] and that fructose – due to the fact that it's metabolized in the liver – doesn't need insulin to be pushed into the cells,[20] which is probably why higher intakes of fructose have been found to improve – yes, improve[21] – insulin sensitivity.

Bears coming out of hibernation reverse their full-blown diabetic state by eating honey, which is a rich source of fructose.

Scientists also are now presenting evidence that diet is the primary driver of the evolution of the complexity of the primate[22] – and possibly human – brain. Among all studied primates, the frugivores – animals who may be omnivore or herbivore but whose diet consists mainly of raw fruits[23] – have the largest, most complex brains. The sugars in the fruits are literally fueling their brains to grow.

Sugars are the primary fuel for the thyroid gland,[24] and the thyroid gland actually controls the rate at which your body burns calories, aka. metabolic rate.[25] When you eat more simple sugars, your thyroid gland produces more T4 thyroid hormone, and with adequate sugars stored in the liver, your body can easily convert T4 into the active T3 form, which greatly improves energy production and metabolic rate.[20]

If sugars and carbohydrates make us all fat, why in the world have almost all bodybuilders for the last hundred years eaten high-carb diets while getting to extremely low body fat levels?

When you lower your calories in order to lose weight, one of the most powerful compounds that can preserve metabolic rate, is in fact; fructose.[26] It supposedly is the substance most notorious for making us gain weight, but in reality, high fructose foods are typically low in caloric content, have the ability to greatly support metabolic rate,[27] and have a muscle sparing effect.[28]

The liver provides about 70% of our active thyroid hormone, by converting thyroxine to T3, but it can provide this active hormone only when it has adequate glucose.

Eating Sugar Will Help Your Body Fight Inflammation Naturally

With everyone running around yelling about sugar being toxic, it might be difficult to believe that, in fact, sugar actually plays a very important role in your body's natural antioxidant defense system, which helps you fight off free radical damage and inflammation.

Glutathione is your "master antioxidant" in the body and

glucose plays a vitally important role in its production. We have a complex endogenous antioxidant system that is ultimately fueled by glucose.

There is a "pathway" known as the pentose phosphate pathway where glucose supplies reducing power to NADPH, from niacin (Vitamin B3), in the form of hydrogen ions and electrons.

Vitamin B2 is then used by the vital enzyme glutathione reductase to pass this reducing power on to glutathione.

Glutathione, your master antioxidant, is then able to neutralize hydrogen peroxide to water, and neutralize lipid peroxides (free radicals from fatty acids like PUFAs) into hydroxy-fatty acids which are less harmful to the body, while recycling Vitamin C - another important antioxidant.

Vitamin C recycles Vitamin E which is your most important defensive antioxidant against PUFA oxidation.

As you can see, this entire system - and all of glutathione's important roles in the body - from fighting against the accumulation of inflammatory free radical species, to protecting against the degradation of fatty acids in the cell membranes, to cleaning up damage caused by PUFAs, all ultimately depends on the availability and action of glucose... sugar.

Does Cancer Really Prefer Sugar?

I'd like to point out an important truth about cancer, and the roles of sugar and fatty acids in cancer.

This is important for my readers to be aware of, precisely because one of the prevailing mythical mantras that has been repeated ad nauseum over the past 30 years is that cancer is "addicted" to sugar and cannot grow in the absence of glucose.

This could not be further from the truth. And the medical community has known this for well over a decade, and has already accumulated quite a large amount of research to back it up.

This mantra has been one of the main talking points we've all heard from proponents of the ketogenic diet, and has been used to prop up their arguments that "sugar is the devil" however, there is substantial evidence demonstrating that a ketogenic diet itself can rapidly accelerate the growth of cancer cells29 with a common mutation that is found in over 60% of cases of melanoma, 100% of hairy cell leukemia, 10% of colorectal cancer, and 5% of multiple myeloma.

Research published in the journal Cell Metabolism in 2017 demonstrated[29] how this extremely common mutation - V600E - rewires the cancer cells' metabolic preference to that of the ketogenic pathway. It does this in order to create a feedback loop to "pour fuel on the fire" for the cancer cell growth and further proliferation throughout the body.

A common energy source in ketosis is acetoacetate. With V600E, the acetoacetate binds a specific protein (the B-raf protein) which promotes oncogenic activation,[30] which gives the cells distinct advantages in growing faster through potential further mutations, gene amplification, and chromosome rearrangements.

This becomes even scarier when you realize that the cancer literally mutates itself in order to fuel its growth through what you eat. Researchers found that when they fed mice with V600E a high fat ketogenic diet, the tumor growth literally doubled in just 4 weeks. As they put it,

"Consistent with our findings above, we found that treatment with a high-fat diet promoted tumor growth rate, sizes, and masses."

Fat oxidation has been found to promote the survival of cancer cells.[31] This is why I think that it is so important to avoid PUFAs as much as possible, since they are so easily oxidized.

Cancer cells are tricky creatures; they have an uncanny ability to mutate and adapt in order to survive. One way that leukemia cells, for example, work is that they prefer to use fatty acid metabolism in order to inhibit the activity of certain proteins to avoid apoptosis, or programmed cell death. This helps the cells stay alive and proliferate.

Again, the important role of fatty acid oxidation in cancer growth is very well known in scientific circles – the public just isn't as aware. Like Dr. Erin Currie, PhD from the Department of Biochemistry & Biophysics at USCF puts it in her paper entitled, Cellular Fatty Acid Metabolism and Cancer,[32]

"Cellular proliferation, a common feature of all cancers, requires fatty acids for synthesis of membranes and signaling molecules. Here we summarize evidence that limiting fatty acid availability can control cancer cell proliferation."

The important thing to understand when it comes to cancer cells is that blanket ideas such as "cancer is addicted to sugar," or "cancer starves without sugar" are quite simply untrue. Cancers can mutate rapidly and get fuel from many things, even amino acids like glutamine.[33] Therefore, the most prudent way to approach cancer treatment from a dietary perspective is for someone to learn about their cancer specifically and follow what's known as a "precision diet" approach to combat that specific cancer.

It's not a one-size-fits-all argument. All ideas that would say it is, are utterly non-scientific.

Sugar Does Not Cause Fatty Liver Disease

The single most common scapegoat for non-alcoholic fatty liver disease is fructose.

Everyone points the finger without any real evidence. If they've "solved" the issue, then how come incidences of fatty liver disease continue to rise so rapidly, and have more than doubled in children over the last 10 years?[34]

They're missing a key element to the equation.

In reality, fructose has been shown to be protective against hepatic liver problems,[35] and when there's adequate choline[36] in the diet, over-feeding of fructose does not lead to fat accumulation in the liver at all.[37] The problem of fatty-liver disease has nothing to do with fructose, and everything to do with eating too much polyunsaturated fatty-acids (which prevent exportation of liver fat)[38] and lack of choline (which is a necessary micronutrient required in the exportation of fat from the liver).[39]

To avoid fatty liver disease, you must avoid consuming PUFAs while simultaneously making sure that you're not deficient in choline. Choline is the one of the single most common nutrient deficiencies in the United States, with an estimated 92% of the entire population carrying this deficiency.[40]

With the prevalence of PUFAs in our cooking oils - being used at nearly every restaurant and in most packaged foods - alongside a 92% population-wide choline deficiency, it's no wonder that around a whopping 100 million adults in the United States are estimated to have non-alcoholic fatty liver disease[41]... a number that continues to increase every year.

How The Ketogenic Diet Is Hurting Your Thyroid, Damaging Your Hormones, and Stalling Your Fat Loss

It probably seems like you cannot go anywhere these days, especially on Facebook without seeing ads all over the place from juiced up bodybuilders touting how the Keto Diet will make you thin, or from Internet Doctors telling you how you need to follow the Keto Diet for fast weight loss and to buy their ketone supplements in order to do so.

Many of you reading this right now have probably actually purchased those supplements or tried their programs. *(Newsflash: according to a recent February 2018 peer-reviewed study,[42] those Ketone supplements don't actually work for inducing ketosis)*

The Keto Diet is the "diet du' jour" right now - the "IN" thing.

But is it actually healthy?

"A Large Crowd, Few People" - The Keto Diet Doesn't Incorporate Health Into Its Worldview

Any recommendations I make throughout this part of the section will be based on the specific reference point of assuming you want two things:

1. Hormonal Balance
2. No Micronutrient Deficiencies

These are the cornerstones of the true definition of Real Health as defined by the Thermo Diet philosophy of accurate thought around nutrition and health in general.

Why would I assume you want these things?

Well, it's funny you ask...

First off, I personally believe that if somebody is to focus on improving their health, or finding a pattern of eating, training, and living that fits Optimal Health, then the entire pursuit should focus on achieving hormonal balance, and through that, a healthy energy metabolism.

This singular pursuit will keep the human body at optimal health.

No other reference point will. It will keep you cancer free, with no autoimmune diseases, no gut problems, no reproductive problems, and with incredible brain health.

Your body literally will be operating at optimal capacity. This is how I intend to live to be 150 years old.

Most people have NO reference point.

They sling studies around, claiming that because they quoted a study, their argument is scientific.

The problem with this shotgun approach to health optimization is that there is literally ZERO reference point. There is no focus.

Myself - or any other person on Earth - can cherry pick research studies all day long to prove any point. The field of "scientific" research is as tainted, corrupt, and misleading as any other human industry and therefore must be always viewed with a skeptical eye. Researchers are subject to economic realities, biases, and laziness just like any of us. Is it so surprising to realize that research could be misleading or poorly done?

The best way to obtain an objective view is to reject Dogma.

If the masses agree on something, it's typically wrong. I'm not sure why this is the case, but it appears to be an age-old truth, recorded from ancient times when the first philosophers began observing human behavior and it's still just as true now.

My favorite philosopher Baltasar Gracian put it this way in his book A Pocket Mirror For Heroes, **"A large crowd, few people."**

So here's the point.

With respect to the Ketogenic Diet in particular, right now we are looking at this "large crowd" with most of the content you will find all over YouTube, IG, Facebook, blogs etc.

The Idea Of Keto "Feels Good"

Shotgun advice quoting random research, with little to no reference to, or understanding of, the way the human body actually works.

That's why, in this part of the chapter, I'm going to go one layer deeper, and, before discussing research studies around the Ketogenic Diet and its effects on humans, I want to explain to you - the reader - some basic biological truths about a couple key systems the human body relies upon for energy metabolism.

Like I said, these are TRUTHS, facts. It's not speculation, opinion, or "research" - it's biology 101.

None of the "Keto Gurus" out there discuss biology, likely because they don't understand or care to know it. However, human biochemistry will light our path on this journey, precisely because it is the truth, and it can help inform our decisions down the road.

I'll keep things easy to understand too, so no worries. This will not be boring.

The idea of Keto "feels good" and that's why it's become so popular once again. It seems logical. But how logical is it really? Is it based in basic human biology?

What Is The Keto Diet, Actually?

First thing's first, let's define the term Ketogenic Diet.

Tons of people sling the term around, but it seems as though people are bending the definition to fit their own purposes, leading to people using the same term for different protocols, which can be misleading and confusing.

Therefore, it'll be helpful for us to identify and agree upon a definition of the actual term "ketogenic diet" before we dig into this series.

The definition I will be using for Keto Diet is a high fat, moderate protein, and very low carbohydrate diet designed to treat epilepsy in children. The depletion of glucose stores in the body requires the body to switch from glucose metabolism to ketone metabolism, a secondary energy source that proponents claim allows your body to "burn fat for fuel."

However, as we will see shortly, this is a drastic oversimplification of the mechanisms at play.

The Ketogenic Diet was started by a physician named Russell Wilder in 1924 specifically to stop seizures in children. It has been an incredibly effective diet protocol for treating epilepsy, so its therapeutic effectiveness for this reason is not challenged.

Interestingly enough, fasting - not the Ketogenic Diet - has been used since ancient Greece to effectively treat epilepsy. Wilder's original intention was to attempt to replicate the therapeutic benefits of fasting in a dietary protocol. Fasting is quite different from the Keto Diet however, since it's a rejuvenative state. We will get deeper into the differences later on.

Now that we know what the Ketogenic Diet is, let's talk about CO_2 and Oxygen production in the body. This is important, so stick with me here.

A healthy metabolism is essential for overall health and long life. And almost nobody would argue this fact. Your metabolism is the sum of the chemical changes taking place inside your cells to provide your body the energy it needs to perform autonomous life-giving processes.

When cellular metabolism declines, aging accelerates, hormonal functioning suffers, and a wide range of disease states and common annoyances occur, such as stubborn body fat, weight gain, muscle wasting, and insomnia, among other things.

With the accepted importance of a healthy systemic metabolism, it's strange how very few people really know how metabolism functions, and therefore are led down all sorts of rabbit holes with misinformation from people who also don't know anything about it.

Here's what you need to know:

You want your cells to produce more CO2 to increase Oxygen use and energy production.

The Bohr Effect, named after Christian Bohr in 1904, describes the inverse relationship between hemoglobin's oxygen binding affinity and blood pH and CO2 production.

The Bohr Effect allows for enhanced unloading of oxygen in metabolically active peripheral tissues such as exercising skeletal muscle. Increased skeletal muscle activity results in localized increases in the partial pressure of carbon dioxide which in turn reduces the local blood pH.

Because of the Bohr Effect, this results in enhanced unloading of bound oxygen by hemoglobin passing through the metabolically active tissue and thus improves oxygen delivery. Importantly, the Bohr Effect enhances oxygen delivery proportionally to the metabolic activity of the tissue.

As more metabolism takes place, the carbon dioxide partial pressure increases thus causing larger reductions in local pH and in turn allowing for greater oxygen unloading. This is especially true in exercising skeletal muscles which may also release lactic acid that further reduces local blood pH and thus enhances the Bohr Effect.

Here's a nifty chart from Christian Bohr describing this visually.

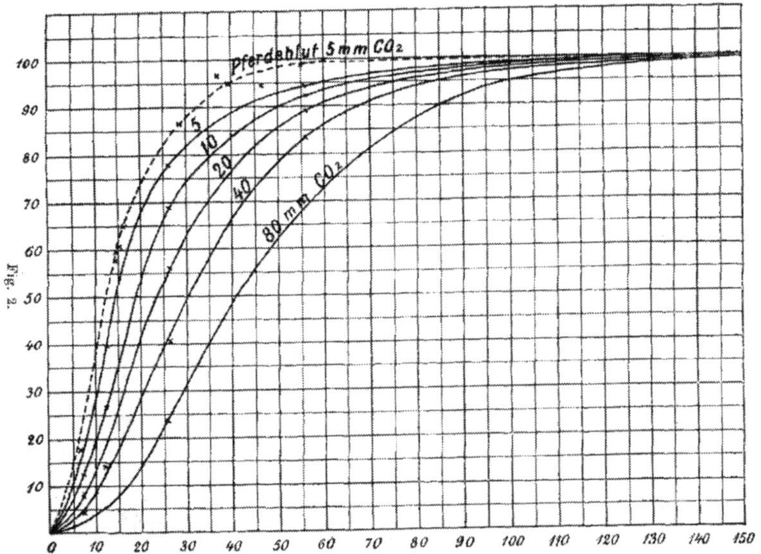

The Haldane Effect describes how oxygenation of blood in the lungs displaces carbon dioxide from hemoglobin which increases the removal of carbon dioxide. Conversely, oxygenated blood has a reduced affinity for carbon dioxide.

Taken together we see that these relationships cause a positive feedback loop, increasing oxygen use and improving metabolic function.

The opposite is also true, as a negative feedback loop. When this system is neglected or abused, and the cells cannot release the oxygen due to lack of CO2, and energy metabolism decreases.

Why does this matter to our understanding of the Keto Diet? I'll show you.

The Randle Cycle, otherwise known as the Glucose Fatty Acid Cycle is characterized by the competition between glucose and fatty acids for their oxidation and uptake in muscle and adipose/fat tissue.

The cycle controls fuel selection and adapts the substrate supply and demand in normal tissues. This cycle adds a nutrient-mediated fine tuning on top of the hormonal control on fuel metabolism. This adaptation to nutrient availability applies to

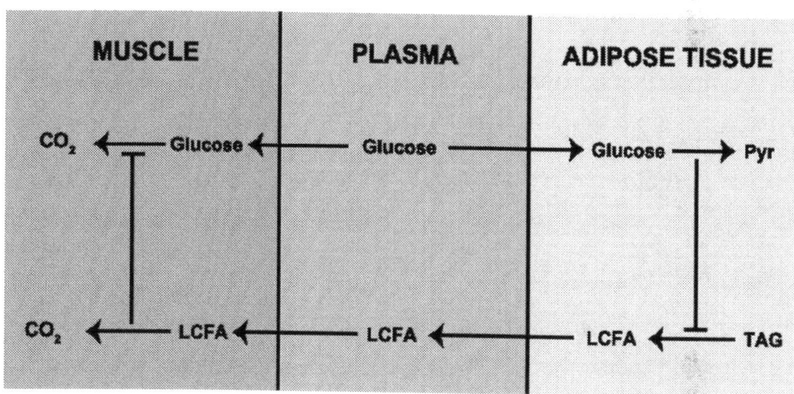

the interaction between adipose tissue and muscle.
So to highlight the important things right now...

1. Carbohydrate breaks down to pyruvate through glycolysis
2. Pyruvate breaks down into the necessary CO2 (remember the Bohr effect) and electrons via the Krebs Cycle
3. The potential energy of electrons produces cellular energy via the electron transport chain

And as we mentioned earlier, when that CO2 production is

optimized, the cells are not just able to increase oxygen use, which leads to a healthier metabolism, but this cycle is also a positive feedback loop.

On a cellular level, this glucose metabolism leads directly to metabolic harmony not just at the cellular level, but also translated to the hormonal level via optimal thyroid functioning, and androgen levels.

Fatty acid metabolism on the other hand occurs via beta oxidation, a slow process that produces much less CO2, therefore less oxygen can be used by the cell, slowing metabolic function in a negative feedback loop. This downward spiral is intended as a survival response, sparing glucose as long as possible, and in the process creating an increasingly poor ability for the body to utilize glucose properly.

This is the Randle Effect, and it explains diabetes. The sugars in the blood cannot be utilized due to fatty acid metabolism shift, because the cells' ability to use glucose is decreasing due to the use of fatty acids, resulting in insulin resistance.

Instead of training cells to use fatty acids for a survival metabolism, this biochemistry would suggest that humans need to utilize carbohydrates for a healthy metabolism and hormonal balance.

Fatty acid metabolism is, and has been, considered secondary and a survival mechanism, and the fact that it's caused by a shift in catecholamine (adrenaline and noradrenaline) stimulation and high cortisol (the body's chief stress hormone) to even achieve the shift from glucose to fatty acid metabolism is not a good sign for those of us seeking hormonal balance, and a healthy metabolism...

The Truth About Ketogenesis: Stress Metabolism At Work

The first thing I want you to understand today is that the current world of "Keto Education" can be super confusing if you're perusing through blogs, videos, and even PubMed. Everyone, even researchers, seem to have a different "opinion" which kinda sucks when you're searching for the truth, right?

So today I'm going to keep things super simple. Because, in the words of Leonardo da Vinci, "Simplicity is the ultimate sophistication."

I want to make sure you, the reader, don't just grasp some simple facts, but you're also able to talk about this subject intelligently in a conversation that will inevitably come up with your friends.

So what is Ketogenesis?

Ketogenesis is simply the production of ketone bodies by the breakdown of fatty acids and ketogenic amino acids.

What is a ketone?

The liver is responsible for making sure that the body (especially the brain and heart) have access to a sufficient supply of energy from the blood. To fulfill that responsibility, it manufactures two energy substrates – glucose and ketones – and exports them into the blood as needed.

The most important ketones are acetoacetic acid and beta-hydroxybutyric acid.

Ketones are water-soluble small molecules. They diffuse throughout the body into cells, and are taken up by mitochondria and oxidized for energy.

Now let's look at how ketogenesis occurs...

The human body prefers a glucose metabolism as a primary energy system, where fatty acid metabolism is considered secondary, reserved for survival situations.
While forced ketogenesis has been shown to have some great therapeutic effects in controlling epilepsy, this special case cannot be assumed healthy across the board, especially since even other therapeutic-related keto diet research shows conflicting evidence. For example, some studies show improvements in cancer control with the keto diet while others show an increase in tumor growth.

In order to flip the "survival switch" from glucose to fatty acid metabolism, the body requires a shift in catecholamine response, and therefore a cortisol increase: the body's chief stress hormone.

Ketosis is inherently stressful on the body.

It is, after all, a survival system designed to preserve your physical body, not necessarily allow it to thrive.

And like I just mentioned, there can be therapeutic benefits of ketosis, these are reserved for special cases where the human body is already deep into a disease state, and does not in any way show evidence for a chronic lifestyle-oriented ketogenic dieting practice.

How The Keto Diet Destroys Your Thyroid Function and Slows Your Metabolism

The Bohr/Haldane Effects and the Randle Cycle demonstrate to us that fatty acid metabolism actually downregulates energy metabolism by decreasing CO_2 production in a negative loop, this shift in catecholamines also damages the thyroid gland.

The thyroid is chiefly responsible for controlling some of the most important hormonal and metabolic processes in your body. Low thyroid hormone levels are also inextricably linked to low androgen production, which leads to not just poor sexual & reproductive function but also other common symptoms such as anxiety, depression, brain fog, insomnia, fat gain, and muscle wasting.

So if this ketone metabolism damages your thyroid by chronically increasing adrenaline, noradrenaline, and cortisol, also suppressing testosterone and other steroid hormone production, then how come some people swear by it? Why do they claim to experience such incredible feelings and "results" during the first 1-3 months on the keto diet?

I'm glad you asked...

Because, funny enough, the increase in fight-or-flight response is precisely *why* they feel an acute increase in focus, energy, "weight loss" and so forth... they're actually putting their body into survival mode, and it's compensating by heightening their awareness, not to mention large scale water flushing gives the impression of quick and easy weight loss and makes the individual feel lighter.

This is a well-known period known as the ***Catecholamine Honeymoon.***

So what's the problem, you might be asking...

Well, you can't rely and an amplification of stress hormones forever. Like I mentioned a minute ago, the heightened stress response eventually starts destroying thyroid function and ravaging your steroid hormone production. It's a unanimously accepted fact that chronically elevated cortisol levels chronically suppress testosterone production.

This is also why many prolonged keto dieters eventually lose all libido and desire for sex. Not to mention experiencing erectile dysfunction in men.

So yeah, stress is not good for our goals...

1. Hormonal balance
2. Fast metabolism

So it looks like another strike against the keto diet.

"You Said Keto Damages Your Thyroid; Can You Elaborate A Bit More On This?"

In this section I want to discuss the basics regarding how a ketogenic diet, or a diet with little to no carbohydrate, can affect your thyroid. By the end of this section you'll have a solid understanding of whether or not the ketogenic diet is recommended for people who have:

1. Hypothyroidism
2. Or want a faster metabolism

Let's get started.

First off, so everyone starts on the same page, I want to make sure you understand what the thyroid gland is.

We all have one, but some of us have healthier ones than others.

The thyroid is one of the most critical hormone-producing glands in the human body. And out-of-whack thyroid can be an absolute nightmare for someone seeking better health and a faster metabolism.

The thyroid hormones regulate vital body functions, including:

- Breathing
- Heart rate
- Central and peripheral nervous systems
- Body weight
- Muscle strength
- Menstrual cycles
- Body temperature
- Cholesterol levels
- Much more!

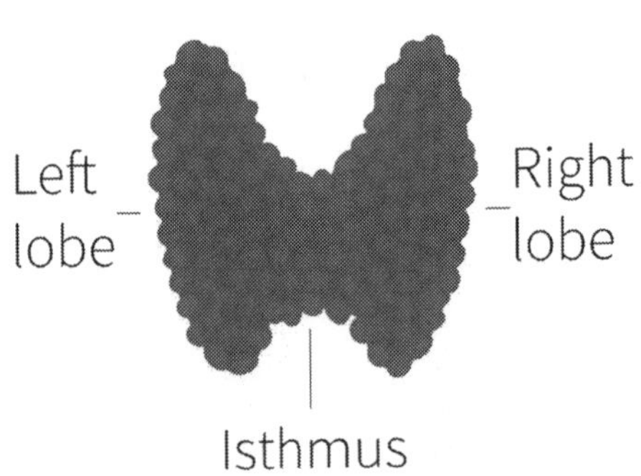

The thyroid gland is about 2-inches long and lies in front of your throat below the prominence of thyroid cartilage sometimes called the Adam's apple. The thyroid has two sides called lobes that lie on either side of your windpipe, and is usually connected by a strip of thyroid tissue known as an isthmus. Some people do not have an isthmus, and instead have two separate thyroid lobes.

How the Thyroid Gland Works

The thyroid is part of the endocrine system, which is made up of glands that produce, store, and release hormones into the bloodstream so the hormones can reach the body's cells. The thyroid gland uses iodine from the foods you eat to make two main hormones:

- Triiodothyronine (T3)
- Thyroxine (T4)

Both of these hormones are extremely important to have balanced, but if you want a healthy metabolism you especially want to increase the amount of T3 conversion. Hypothyroidism, or low functioning thyroid characterized by a slow metabolism, is characterized by less than normal amount of T3 production. Increasing T3 will help to solve hypothyroidism.

So where do carbohydrates fit into this?

Thyroid hormones are essential to maintain and regulate carbohydrate/energy metabolism.[43]
Conversely, the energy (glucose) we get from carbs is required to fuel the production of thyroid hormones.

This is because the parts of the brain ultimately responsible for thyroid hormone regulation – the hypothalamus and the pituitary gland – require glucose to function.

In fact, the main regulation hormone, called Thyroid Stimulating Hormone (TSH), is made up partly of glucose molecules.[44]

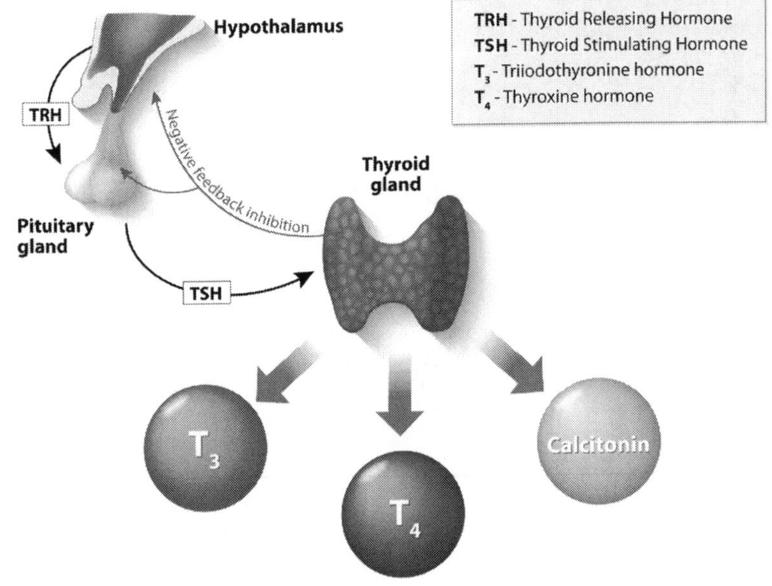

In addition to these important roles, carb intake appears to influence the amount of T3 that gets converted from T4 thyroid hormone. This is important for hypothyroidism as T3 is the active thyroid hormone that you need to increase.

It appears that when carb intake is drastically reduced, conversion of T3 from T4 declines.[45]

This could be explained by the possible interaction between insulin and the enzymes that convert T4 into the T3.[46]

So to sum it up nicely: Thyroid hormones rely on glucose for production and conversion, especially the conversion of T3 from T4.

Now let's talk about survival mechanisms.

The body naturally will downregulate metabolism through this pathway when it goes into a survival mode, physiologically... for example, extreme prolonged calorie restriction and long water fasts, will both cause the body to slow metabolic function, shuttling resources toward vital organs.

The ketogenic diet was originally designed, for therapeutic reasons in epileptic patients, with the intention of mimicking fasting on a physiological level.[47]

One of the key differences between fasting and the keto diet is that water fasts are typically only done for short acute periods of time, for example 1-3 days, or in very extreme cases up to 30 days for people healing their bodies of cancers or autoimmune diseases - and water fasts are typically used as a means of healing and rejuvenation, since the body does not need to focus any energy on digestion and can focus on complete systemic rest.

The keto diet on the other hand, since people are consuming and digesting calories, puts people into this physiological state for months to years at a time, therefore putting the body under a significant amount of physiological stress.

One of the manifestations of this long term stress response is a drastic slowing of thyroid - and therefore, metabolic - functioning. T3 conversion slows down significantly.

A number of small scale studies[48] have shown that after a period of starvation, refeeding with carbohydrates[49] – but not with protein or fats – normalised thyroid hormone levels.[50]
In one of the studies, researchers evaluated the effects of restricting carbs at various levels (85, 44 and 2% of total energy intake) on thyroid hormones in healthy male participants.

Results found that the high carbohydrate diet had no impact, whereas the very low carbohydrate diet did. It caused decreased T3 levels, increased rT3 and free T4 levels.[48]

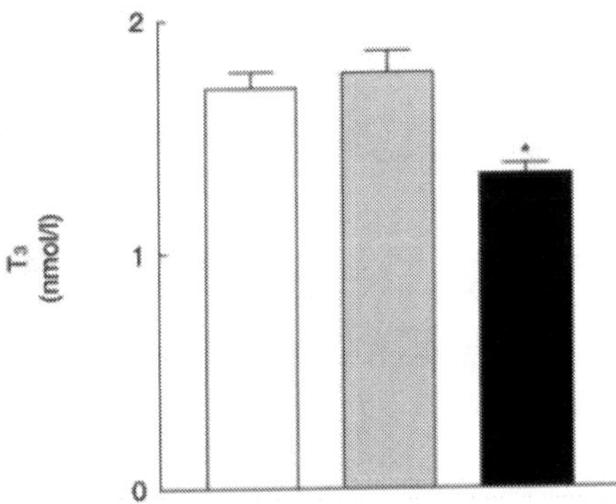

*Average T3 plasma concentrations after 11 days of high carbohydrate diet (white), control diet (grey) and low carbohydrate diet (black) in the healthy males. The * indicates a significantly lower T3 level for the low carbohydrate diet, which is not desirable in hypothyroidism.*

These results are similar to those of another study where participants either fasted or received an 800 Kcal low calorie diet consisting of either 0%, 25% or 100% carbohydrate, for a period of 2 weeks.

The results showed T3 levels were reduced from both fasting and the 0% carbohydrate diet, but not from the 100% carbohydrate diet.[45]

It would seem that, from a systemic view of the endocrinology and biochemistry at play here, that the ketogenic diet downregulates thyroid function due to decreased TSH through the hypothalamic-pituitary axis, as well as decreased conversion of T3 from T4 thyroid hormone, which can either make hypothyroidism worse, or cause it in a formerly healthy person.

Hopefully this is helpful information for anyone on the fence in considering whether or not the keto diet craze is healthy for their thyroid function.

More Keto Research:

Beyond biochemistry basics that I've already presented, there is a literal mountain of peer-reviewed research to support the claims I am making. I didn't just make this all up for fun, I actually read all of this research to come to my conclusions...

The Keto Diet Hurts Physical Performance and Exercise

<u>Capacity</u>

This study states that there is no evidence high fat and low carb diets enhance training.[51]

This study[52] shows that low carb dieting decreases performance in supramaximal exercise due to decreased glycolytic activity and an increase in resting sympathoadrenal system post workout.

This study[53] shows that high protein low carb dieting leads to metabolic acidosis.

This study[54] confirms that Ketosis does not have any advantageous effect on performance in athletes.

This study[55] shows a decrease in glycolysis even in the presence of adequate glycogen in a ketogenic state.

This shows that the keto diet decreased the amount of time to exhaustion,[56] and a decrease in energy and were unable to easily undertake high bouts of exercise.

This study[57] shows that the keto diet is not ideal for athletes. This study[58] shows negation of performance in endurance athletes.

This study[59] shows ketosis does impair performance due to lack of carb intake but say that inuit people who ancestrally eat keto have no impairment in performance.

And despite keto gurus touting how good the diet is for focus, the research shows a decline in physical and cognitive performance.[60]

<u>**Eat Fat To Burn Fat? Not True...**</u>

This study shows after six months there was no decrease in weight.[61] So much for weight loss.

This study[62] showed keto dieters having no measurable difference in fat free mass.

This study[63] showed that the body composition difference was consistent with diet and less caloric intake not due to low intake of carbs.

While this shows[64] weight loss was directly related to decrease in calories not low carb intake.

This states[65] that low fat dieting is more effective for fat loss and weight maintenance than low carb.

This study[66] shows a significant difference in weight loss due to water loss in keto state.

This demonstrates that a high fat diet can result in significant changes in gut microbial composition, alter gut bacterial composition, and promote obesity.[67] This study also shows alteration of gut microbiota and causing more likeliness to obesity due to a high fat diet.[68]

Keto Actually Makes Insulin Resistance Worse (Proof)

This study[69] shows dysfunction with a GLUT transporter causing malabsorption of glucose.

This study shows that ketotic state induced by the EKD nitrogen balance was decreased initially, serum lipids were not pathologically elevated, and blood glucose oxidation at rest was reduced while the subjects remained euglycemic.[70]

This study[71] shows an increase in non-oxidative glucose disposal.

This study[72] shows how the keto diet causes insulin resistance formation in high fat fed mice.

Confirmed again: High fat feeding leads to insulin resistance.[73]

High fat diet leads to insulin independent diabetes.[74] Increased lipid oxidation leads to glucose intolerance.[75]

Increases in free fatty acids lead to increased symptoms in undesirable insulin response.[76]

Free fatty acids reduce responsiveness to glucose dependent insulin secretion.[77]

High sucrose diet does not cause negative effects towards inducing diabetes.[78]

The Ketogenic Diet Causes Micronutrient Deficiencies

This study[79] shows acid producing diets like the keto diet are detrimental and this diet ends in decreased B12 and folic acid intake. Due to lack of vitamin D in the keto diet the researchers found that there was bone mineral deficiency in the subjects of this study.[80]

This study[81] states the true keto diet causes a lack of protein and therefore growth.

This study[82] shows that the keto diet has to be supplemented with minerals, and has a specific lack of selenium.

While this study[83] shows a decrease in glycine and a couple of other really important anti-stress amino acids when on keto.

How To Transition Back To Eating Carbohydrates After Trying Keto

Over the past few years as I have been testing out this dietary philosophy with my friends, family, and in our 1500 person Thermo beta group, one of the most common situations people find themselves in is transitioning from the keto diet back to a more sustainable and healthy way of eating on Thermo.

Eating Thermo is quite simple for somebody who is eating carbohydrates regularly but who just needs to do some tweaks like change their carb sources and stop consuming PUFAs.

However, we've learned in the research that eating "Keto" for prolonged periods of time actually worsens insulin resistance in the body, essentially making people diabetic, so when people try to transition back to eating carbs, there may be a period of time where the dietary changes make their body react poorly.

For example, eating starch again might make their blood sugar swing wildly again throughout the day.

This is only because eating a ketogenic diet essentially trained their body to not be able to use insulin properly, while heightening their adrenaline and cortisol chronically, so for anybody who finds themselves in this scenario, just know that you will need a period of about 2-4 weeks to reacclimate and bring your body back to a state of balance.

Through testing protocols on people, I've found the following protocol to be most effective for facilitating this transition.

- Eat within a 6-8 hour eating window every day. Outside of that eating window consume nothing but water or organic coffee. The fasting will not only help keep your blood sugar more steady through the day, it will improve your insulin sensitivity naturally as you make this transition.

- Break your fast with 1-2 pieces of organic fruit and 1-2 cups of grass fed bone broth. Another option is to break your fast with a smoothie made with organic fruits and a scoop of collagen protein.
- While other people deeper into Thermo can usually enjoy quite large carbohydrate-rich meals (from Thermo sources) with no blood sugar issues at all, you will require some time to get that point, so I recommend keeping your portions of Thermo-approved carbohydrates during your meal to a moderate to small size.
- Focus your meals on eating high quality meats and fats from non-PUFA sources alongside this small portion of starchy carbohydrates
- Do not snack, just eat your planned 2-3 meals during this 6-8 hour eating window, including the smoothie or bone broth/fruit meal to break the fast
- Walk for 30-60 minutes outdoors every day. Inactivity has been found to increase insulin resistance.[84-86]

As the first few weeks develop, you will find that your body can much more easily handle carbohydrate consumption. You will begin to truly feel as though energy jumps back into your system.

As you begin feeling better, start to experiment with less overall fat intake, making up those calories from Thermo-approved carbohydrates.

CHAPTER FOUR

DON'T EAT PUFAS

THE LAW OF TOXIC OILS

It is time to expose one of the biggest health scams in history. Polyunsaturated fats, also known as PUFAs, are toxic to the human body, destroying your thyroid's ability to function properly and lowering your reproductive hormone levels, causing sexual dysfunction and hormonal imbalance. The weak double bond structure of the fatty acid chains in PUFAs leads to easy oxidation from exposure to air, sunlight, and body heat - causing the rapid production of free radicals, which impact the structure and function of human DNA and cells. These rancid oils are currently found in almost every household in the Western world, and used for high-heat cooking! Currently, most people believe that these "vegetable oils" are "heart healthy" alternatives to using animal fats or fruit fats, however this couldn't be further from the truth. PUFA-based cooking oils originally started off as a toxic chemical byproduct from industrial usages, thrown away as waste. However, due to profiteering propaganda and bribery of the American Heart Association, these oils quickly made their way into the food supply of hundreds of millions of people, to the extreme detriment of the health of the entire population. If you remember only one thing from reading this book it should be this: stop eating PUFAs.

The late 1800s and early 1900s set the stage for quite possibly the biggest corruption of our public health to-date.

"What was garbage in 1860, was fertilizer in 1870, cattle feed in 1880, and table food and many things else in 1890," reported Popular Science[1] about the evolution of the waste product cottonseed oil and how it steadily made its way to become a dietary staple in American society, alongside a host of other "vegetable oils."

This tale of two profiteering businessmen, William Procter and James Gamble, and the perfect storm of how they found a chemical waste product and sold it to the public, is one of the most disturbingly impressive marketing case studies of the last century.

Soap was once widely made using animal fats and sold in large wheels or chunks that the consumer could use to break pieces off when needed. Procter & Gamble, brothers-in-law and business partners just beginning their journey to build one of the world's largest consumer products companies, that obviously still exists today, decided that they would like to engineer a soap that achieved two things for the consumer:

1. It needed to be packaged as an individual-sized "bar" of soap – instead of having to break off ugly chunks of soap, now the customer would be able to buy a conveniently sized single bar of soap. This made the economics of selling soap far more profitable, and turned a somewhat homemade or artisanal product into a new, marketable household item that could be sold with flashy packaging via convincing new advertisements.
2. It needed to float – soap made with animal fats was heavy enough to sink in the bathtub, leaving the bathing individual to flounder around in the soapy water trying to find the lost soap. Procter & Gamble had the idea that they needed to find a way to make the soap float so the consumer could easily keep track of it.

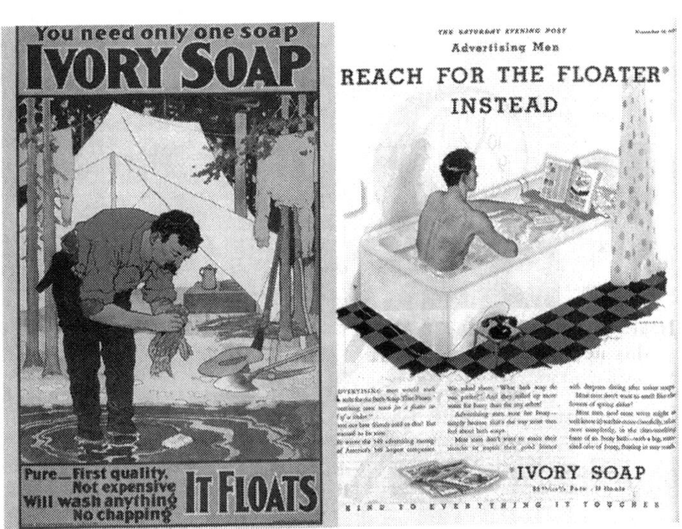

In order to achieve both of these criteria simultaneously, they came up with the idea to use a different type of fat in the soap recipe. Instead of the heavy animal fats, they had their first "floating" success with using coconut oil and palm oil.

However, since these oils are not native crops to the United States, importing them was unnecessarily expensive. The creative businessmen came up with another new idea.

Cottonseed oil.

To that point, cottonseed oil was seen purely as a waste byproduct of cotton farming, and the oil itself was dumped into rivers.

Procter & Gamble started buying up the oil for next to nothing, since - after all - it was just waste to that point - and used it to make their new floating bars of soap. The soap, still known as Ivory Soap, was a massive success.

With their newfound "natural resource" of cottonseed oil in abundance and their marketing prowess, they hired a German chemist by the name of Edwin Kayser who created a new process to turn the liquid cottonseed oil into a "creamy, pearly white substance" that resembled lard - this process became known as hydrogenation.

At that time, lard was widely used for cooking in the average household. Their newly engineered cottonseed oil substance was poised to compete with the massive market share that lard and other animal fats held as cooking fats in every American household.

Procter & Gamble named their franken oil, Crisco.

They claimed that the name Crisco conjured up ideas of "crispness, freshness, and cleanliness."[2]

To market Crisco, they hired an advertising agency, the J. Walter Thompson Agency, who undertook one of the largest marketing campaigns of that century by sending Crisco samples to the "influencers" of that era, nutritionists, chefs, grocers, and restaurant owners. Samples of foods cooked with Crisco were given out on the streets for free to demonstrate just how good the food would taste when the customer chose Crisco over traditional cooking fats.

Special bonuses were also given out to people who purchased Crisco, such as cookbooks specifically designed with recipes only using Crisco.

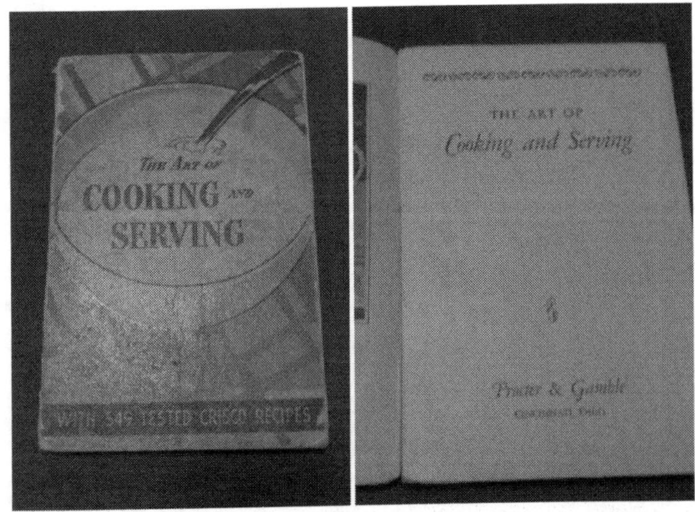

The campaign against animal fats had begun in earnest.

Procter & Gamble even went so far as to bribe the American Heart Association for $1.5M to publicly endorse Crisco. Abusing their public trust, and using the guise of "science," the AHA launched a smear campaign against saturated fats by claiming that they caused heart disease and raised levels of "bad" cholesterol in the body.

Crisco, however, was the savior. The "heart healthy" choice for Americans.

As this dogmatic propaganda steadily spread over the 1900s, the US government got involved, launching public health initiatives such as the 1977 Dietary Guidelines for Americans which denounced saturated fats, while the Center For Science In The Public Interest (CSPI) publicly recommended that all Americans should switch from saturated fats to hydrogenated oils.

Collusion with public interest groups turned out to be an extremely effective marketing strategy for Procter & Gamble, leading to not just hundreds of millions of dollars in sales of Crisco, but also development of new "innovative" cooking oils and competitor companies using safflower oil, canola oil, sunflower seed oil, corn oil, flaxseed oil, rapeseed oil, and many others - along with the widespread popularity of another franken oil - margarine.

Beyond the fact that the invention of these oils was purely

novel, and the fact that the way they have been marketed to us as "heart healthy options" is purely unethical and untrue, one thing rings true above the conspiratorial fog: all of these oils are extremely toxic to the human body and their presence in our diets has likely correlated with the massive rise in hypothyroidism, obesity, diabetes, and all manner of other metabolic and hormonal disorders across our entire population over the last 100 years.

PUFAs Destroy Human Health

The main type of fatty acid in vegetable oils is what is known as a polyunsaturated fatty acid. It is an easily oxidized fat that is extremely toxic to the human body and can cause a whole host of health problems.

This is a well known fact in scientific research circles, however... something is amiss...

Search around the web for a couple minutes and you'll find a lot of articles (many of which from government sponsored sources and "official" western medical associations) touting how good PUFAs are for you.

The interesting thing is though, they're all fluff. In fact, this is Propaganda 101. Like I mentioned before, the collusion with public interest groups and scientists on the so-called health benefits of PUFAs has been widespread for over 100 years.

Back in Chapter 3, I also mentioned how the Burr laboratory findings were used as scientific fodder to prop up the idea that these oils are "essential" to the human body. Nothing could be further from the truth.

However, the dogma is still alive and strong, with major medical associations and even institutions like Harvard continuing to publish material to endorse the consumption of these toxic oils.

For example, on this government-sponsored website[3] they explicitly tell you to substitute saturated fats in your cooking with corn oil, soy oil, and safflower oil - all PUFA-laden vegetable oils that are terrible for your body.

Again, on Webmd the website recommends using **more** PUFAs in our diets.[4]

Even the American Heart Association recommends that we consume more PUFA in our diets.[5] SHAPE magazine doctors recommend that one third of our entire daily caloric intake comes from PUFAs.[6]

Harvard tells us that PUFAs are better for us than saturated fats.[7]

The list goes on and on and on[8] with these "health authorities" telling the masses to keep consuming more and more PUFAs in our diets. Heck, even the American Diabetes Association tells diabetics to eat more PUFAs (there is a massive amount of evidence demonstrating that PUFAs actually CAUSE diabetes).[9]

It seems we are living in the "upside down" world where Lies are called truth and the real Truth is concealed from the public.

It's time we take our health back. I'm happy to lead the way...

Most if not all of these claims on polyunsaturated fats being healthy are for the simple fact that the polyunsaturated fats lower the levels of the so called bad cholesterol which is LDL cholesterol.

What is Polyunsaturated Fat and What Makes It Different From Other Types Of Fat?

Polyunsaturated fat is a molecule that has the same molecular structure as the rest of the fats that exist with a carboxyl group on one end connected to a chain of carbon atoms that have hydrogen atoms attached to them, all of the carbon have two hydrogen molecules attached except for the middle two they only have on the same side of the molecule.

The "unsaturated" portion of the molecular structure is a double bond that forms between one or in the case of a polyunsaturated fat two or more carbon atoms.

Monounsaturated fats have the exact same structure but with only one double bond in between two of the carbon atoms hence the beginning of the word "Mono" meaning one.

Saturated fats have the exact same molecular structure with a carboxyl group on one end and a chain of carbon atoms with attached hydrogen atoms. The thing that makes them different however is the fact that they have no double bonds between any of the carbon atoms.

Finally we have trans fats. These fats should be avoided in all circumstances. These fats have the same structure with the double bonds (either a single double bond or multiple) except with a carboxyl group on the other end of the molecule and instead of having a chain of carbon atoms with hydrogen attached straight across they have one of the middle hydrogen molecules on the opposite side of the molecule, on the "trans side."

The Top Common Food Sources of Polyunsaturated Fats

PUFA can be found in trace amounts of many foods, even in land animals in varying concentrations, mostly depending on their diet.

Livestock being fed corn and soy will have much higher PUFA concentration in their fat tissue than lifetime grass fed and finished livestock, for example. This is why it's very important to pay close attention to the quality of the meat you consume.

However, there are plenty of foods that are very high in PUFA that I recommend you eliminate from your diet completely. These are namely:

- Vegetable oils of all varieties: safflower oil, flaxseed oil, sunflower seed oil, any nut based oil, canola oil, rapeseed oil, corn oil, peanut oil, rice bran oil, cottonseed oil
- Frankenstein cooking oils: margarine, Crisco, or anything similar being marketed under a different guise in the grocery store
- Nuts and seeds
- Fish oil supplements

Yes, unfortunately fish oil supplements are not what you think they are either, despite heavy marketing telling you that they are a panacea of health. It is nearly impossible to consume fish oil without it already being rancid by the time it gets to your home.

Heat and light are well-known oxidizers of PUFA, and the fish oil processing, packaging, and shipping lifecycle exposes the supplements to plenty of heat and light, with the bottles usually transported in 120 degree F trucks, among plenty of other exposures.

However, in the off chance it isn't rancid yet, research has proven to us that fish oil will auto-oxidize when consumed due to body temperature.[10] Your natural body heat is hot enough to easily rancidize the oil upon contact. Fish oils are well-known in the research to form harmful oxidative byproducts through free radical pathways, therefore I recommend avoiding them.[11]

The Essential Fatty Acid Myth

If you recall from the story in the introduction to the chapter on sugar, the origin story of how the "essential fatty acid" hypothesis came to be is quite tenuous to say the least.

Even in the face of contrary evidence - actually, quite literally opposite evidence - Dr. Burr ignored the conflicting findings in his lab and pushed through with the invention of his fake disease "essential fatty acid deficiency."

It has been used since then to prop up non-scientific arguments for the PUFA-laden oils that have poisoned our population in the meantime.

If this seems like a strong claim to you, please consider the fact that actual research supports this claim as well.

Researchers have found that when they measure the effects of an "EFA deficiency" - or rather the absence of these "essential" fatty acids in the human diet, you actually see a marked improvement in inflammation, diabetes, and resistance to endotoxin in the body.

These findings are perfectly in line with what we know according to the body of research demonstrating that PUFAs are inflammatory, cause insulin resistance, lower defenses to endotoxin, damage thyroid function, and cause hormonal imbalance.

For example, in one study comparing an EFA deficient diet to a diet high in EFAs, the researchers found that EFA deficiency improved many important biomarkers of fighting inflammation in the body (they seemed a bit surprised by this).[12]

Another study found that EFA deficient rats became highly resistant to endotoxin in their bodies, but this defense vanished with the reintroduction of EFAs, leaving them open and susceptible to endotoxin only after consuming the fatty acids again.[13]

And again, multiple studies have shown both improvements[14] and prevention of diabetes by lowering the consumption of EFAs in the body.[15]

The idea that these fatty acids are somehow "essential" to our health is nothing more than propaganda - false dogma that has been spread through the last 100 years due to special interest profiteering.

There's no need to believe in this lie any longer.

PUFA Is Toxic For Human Consumption: Why You Should Avoid It Like The Plague

What happens when you eat polyunsaturated fats?

The higher temperature from our bodies causes the rigid double bonds found in the molecule to be oxidized and broken apart because they are not flexible and able to withstand the heat.

When this happens the molecule forms free radicals which are molecular structures that contain an unpaired electron.

Basically when this happens the free radical goes around wreaking havoc on all the other molecules around it to find a way to either gain an electron or get rid of an extra electron. In the process of trying to do this, it damages other healthy molecular structures when polyunsaturated fats are oxidized which in turn damages healthy cells and vital structures that are needed to perform optimally.

This also happens to monounsaturated fats but on a lower level because they only have one double bond making them a little more flexible giving them a higher smoke point, which is why consuming them is okay in small amounts.

Then there are saturated fats, the fats that don't have and double bonds. This allows the fat molecule to be really flexible allowing it to have the best stability out of all the fatty acids.

These single bonds are able to move and rotate in whatever way they need to, allowing them to adapt to high temperatures very well. This allows the fats to be consumed by the average human being without the oxidation of the fatty acid creating free radicals.

This NIH-backed study demonstrates the fact of how double bond content of PUFAs negatively correlates with mammal lifespan.[16] The more PUFA you consume, the shorter the lifespan.

This study[17] demonstrates how PUFAs cause disruption in normal cell membrane structure.

Here's Why Every Single Pro-PUFA Argument Cites "Cholesterol" And Why Their Arguments Are All Completely Inaccurate

In fact, it actually seems to me to be a bit shady how all these organizations are propping up a false narrative of cholesterol being the bad guy, and using shill scientists and doctors to support the narrative.

One thing that I find interesting is that people don't even realize that HDL and LDL are not even the actual cholesterol molecules that are the so-called "bad guys."

HDL (High Density Lipoprotein) and LDL (Low Density Lipoprotein) are simply lipoproteins which are carrier proteins for the cholesterol to get from point A to point B.[18]

HDL transports excess cholesterol to the liver where it can be excreted by the body.[19] LDL transports cholesterol to cells throughout the body to be used to make steroid hormones and other things like the cell membrane.

The problem that many had with LDL cholesterol was the implication that it builds up in the arteries "causing" heart disease.

This is a *false idea* because the reality is that when there is damage in the artery the LDL cholesterol is sent to the damaged area of the artery to give those cells the cholesterol they need to properly heal themselves, but when the LDL is in excess there is too much of a good thing in one area.

Cholesterol is not the bad guy. Please stop believing that myth. In fact, the medical journal the Expert Review of Clinical Pharmacology recently released a comprehensive review of the literature and their discussion states that "LDL-C does not cause heart disease" citing the fact that after close analysis of all the available research on the subject, there is not enough evidence to link LDL cholesterol to causing heart disease.

Their explicit conclusion sums this up nicely, *"Our search for falsifications of the cholesterol hypothesis confirms that it is unable to satisfy any of the Bradford Hill criteria for causality and that the conclusions of the [authors of other reviews endorsing the hypothesis] are based on misleading statistics, exclusion of unsuccessful trials and by ignoring numerous contradictory observations."*

Accurate Research Tells A Completely Different Story About PUFAs and Vegetable Oils That The "Powers That Be" Don't Want

This study[17] had a negative correlation between the maximum longevity of mammals and double bond content. Their claim was

"These results, together with previous ones obtained in rodents, birds, and humans, suggest that the low degree of tissue fatty acid unsaturation of longevous homeothermic animals could have been selected during evolution to protect the tissues against oxidative damage."

This study showed that when the mothers consumed a high level of PUFA while pregnant that the concentration of PUFA caused an increase in the estrogen signal for the mothers and a decrease in the progesterone signaling.[20]

This study[21] supports that the higher the PUFA intake the lower the MLSP or the Maximum lifespan for mammals was saying "MLSP indeed decreases as the ratio of n-3 to n-6 PUFAs increases."

This study[22] showed that the polyunsaturates exposed to neural tissue of embryonic chicks during various stages of development could impair neural development.

They also stated that glucagon naturally suppressed mobilisation within the fetus. Stating

"For example, at day 18 of development, the proportions (% w/w of fatty acids) of 20:5n-3 and 22:6n-3 released into the incubation medium were respectively 6.5 and 7.5 times higher than in the

original tissue TAG. Glucagon stimulated the overall rate of mobilisation by approx. 2-fold and also partially suppressed the preferential mobilisation of C20-22 polyunsaturates."

This study[23] showed that the consumption of PUFA (arachidonic acid, eicosapentaenoic acid) in a dose dependent manner increased the vascular permeability of the vascular system within the brain in rats by the increase of free radical damage caused by the breakdown of the fatty acids.

This study[24] showed the effect of DHA, EPA, and ALA on the electrophysiological effects of the heart. The results showed that all of them had some kind of negative inotropic (speed of contraction) and chronotropic (speed of rate) effects. The EPA and ALA actually elongated the QTc interval as well. The higher the concentration the more spread out the wave intervals were on the QTc.

This study[25] shows that there is a direct inverse correlation between the amount of total daily energy consumption coming from polyunsaturated fatty acids and testosterone production.

In a dose dependent manner the more of the total energy consumption of fat came from PUFA the lower the testosterone became. This study also had good findings with high amounts of protein having a negative correlation to testosterone as well.

This study[26] states the prevalence of an increased omega 6 diet and its prevalence towards increasing hyperinsulinemia and insulin resistance. It also refers to the increased prevalence of free radicals with the increased PUFA consumption.

This study[27] concludes that the Omega-6 fatty acids are related to increased inflammation through various mechanisms.

This study[28] was very interesting, showing that a diet rich in omega 6 fatty acids during pregnancy (lactation and gestation) of mice had a positive correlation with Autistic Sociability Disorder. They correlate it to the increased stress that is caused during the pregnancy period.

This study[29] looks at the effects of polyunsaturated fatty acids on neonatal monocytes. The claims are that the polyunsaturated fatty acids modulate the immune response in vitro.

This study[30] showed the prevalence of unsaturated fatty acids having an atherogenesis effect. This was due to the high metabolization of HDL cholesterol, and the impairment of the ABCA1 macrophage pathway.

This study[31] showed the prevalence of the high omega 6-omega 3 ratio as seen in the typical western diet is correlated with increased risk of heart disease. Autoimmune disease, cancer, and inflammatory diseases. The authors go into detail about how an increase in the omega 3 content of the diet reduces the risk of these diseases and all cause mortality.

This study[32] showed that there was a positive correlation

between men who were on a vegetarian diet (which is naturally higher in PUFA) and SHBG, versus those that were on an Omnivorous diet had significantly less. The conclusion was that the vegetarian group of men (higher PUFA diet) had significantly less testosterone available for the androgen receptor sites.

This study[33] talked about LDL oxidation and the effect that it can have an effect on general signaling pathways and gene expression. Also talks a bit about the apoptosis effect in the epithelial cells in the arterial walls by the oxidative damage.

This study[34] talks about 5 different commercial solvents that are used for extraction of cottonseed oil. The solvents include hexane, benzene, acetone, ethyl-ether, and Buta-none.

This study[35] showed that the ingestion of omega 3 fatty acid when oxidized increased inflammation specifically in the upper part of the digestive tract and the duodenum.

This study[36] shows the effect of consumption of Omega 3 fatty acids specifically DHA and the susceptibility it has in the peroxidation of cell membranes and the inhibiting effect it has on the antioxidant system.

This study[37] showed the effect of EPA consumption of young males and the fact that it decreased fibrinolytic activity and increased coagulation activity. Their claim came to show that daily EPA consumption could affect the liver and kidney functioning.

This study[38] showed a direct link between polyunsaturated fatty acids and reduced function of the exportation of fats out of the liver from regulation of hepatic apolipoprotein B degradation and VLDL production.

This study[39] was significant in showing how statins and vegetable oils decreased survival rates in rats that were prone to stroke and spontaneous hypertension. Shows the relationship that these oils damage kidneys, and inhibit many vitamin K2 pathways.

This was a huge study[40] that showed the association of PUFA intake and the relevancy of IBS, Crohns, and Ulcerative Colitis. The study had over 4000 controls.

This study[41] showed a correlation between wound healing and topical treatment of polyunsaturated fats. It showed that the omega 3 fatty acid linolenic acid significantly delayed wound healing and delayed nitric oxide production at the wound site.

This study[42] showed that there might be an inverse correlation towards early memory in pre-birth infants and early exposure to PUFA.

This study[43] shows how PUFA causes an efflux of calcium ions from the mitochondria inhibiting the function of the mitochondria.

This study[44] showed the effect of PUFA exposure (as well as a derivative of PUFA) and alteration of steroidogenesis and an increase on glucocorticoids from the adrenals.There was also a stimulation of adrenocorticotropic hormone ACTH.

"But I Thought PUFAs Were Good For Me, and Saturated Fat Was Bad?!"

Like I mentioned earlier, we seem to be living in some kind of Upside Down from Stranger Things... a world where everything is backwards, and lies are masquerading as truth.

In fact, saturated fats (SFA) are very good for men and women who want to optimize their hormones naturally and quickly to bring their bodies back into balance and experience incredible natural transformations and healing.

This article[45] supports the fact that there is no correlation between SFA and all-cause mortality, coronary heart disease, CHD mortality, ischaemic stroke, or type 2 diabetes in healthy adults.

It also states that greater consumption of SFA was linked to slower generation of atherosclerosis, while PUFA and Carb intake (most likely carb-heavy foods combined with high PUFA concentration) were linked to an increased progression.

This study[46] showed that the saturated fatty acids suppressed adrenocorticotropic hormone release induced by stimulation with corticotropin-releasing hormone in the pituitary.

This study[47] shows a positive correlation between SFA and testosterone levels.

This study[48] showed a positive correlation between coconut oil consumption as well as pig lard and testosterone levels rising significantly more versus those that were on a diet containing olive oil, fish oil, sunflower oil, and sesame oil.

Other Dangerous Issues With Vegetable Oils

As research around fats continues to surface, we are now aware of the true health impacts that occur from consuming hydrogenated vegetable oils. These oils have other troublesome properties that can lead to both acute and chronic health concerns.

Manufacturers Add Harmful Ingredients to Vegetable Oil

Consumers who purchase vegetable oils often assume that the bottle simply contains oil from vegetables. Unfortunately, this is not the case. Manufacturers add a host of hidden, harmful ingredients, and "vegetable" oil is a misnomer since none of the oils are actually made from vegetables at all - but rather various kinds of seeds or other cheap crops like soy and corn.

Genetically Modified Organisms (GMOs)

Between 85-90% of conventional soybean, corn, cotton and canola oils are grown from GMO seeds.[49] Although the research is still in the early stages on the impact of genetically modified ingredients to human health, The Institute for Responsible Technology reports that animal studies found genetically modified foods cause "organ damage, gastrointestinal and immune system disorders, accelerated aging, and infertility." The Institute further states that when GMOs were introduced in 1996, "the percentage of Americans with three or more chronic illnesses jumped from 7% to 13% in just 9 years; food allergies skyrocketed, and disorders such as autism, reproductive disorders, digestive problems, and others are on the rise."[50]

BHA and BHT

Butylated Hydroxyanisole (BHA) and Butylated Hydroxytoluene (BHT) are also added to the vegetable oils to keep them "fresh" and prevent spoilage. These artificial ingredients have led to cancer, have suppressed the immune system, led to infertility, kidney and liver damage and behavioral problems.

The Processing of Vegetable Oil Creates Dangerous Chemicals

Now that we've covered how vegetable oils came to be so common in our food supply, if you're not disturbed enough by that information then let's take a look at how they're actually processed.

While some vegetable oils are cold-pressed, a minimal technique that leaves many of its original nutrients, this practice is not common. Most cooking oil is heavily processed to create a clear and pleasant oil,[51] and "go through an insane amount of processing with chemical solvents, steamers, neutralizers, de-waxers, bleach and deodorizers before they end up in the bottle."

> *"At first, vegetable seeds are diskinned and dehulled and crushed into coarse meal. They are then heated to extract the oil from the meal. In addition to the heat, up to 20,6850 kilopascals of pressure is used on the meal to extract as much oil as possible."*
> *— Corn Refiners Association*

But that's not all — hydrocarbon and neurotoxin hexane solvents are then added for maximum extractions. Hexane is a byproduct that's created during the production of gasoline, which is hazardous to our health and pollutes our air with toxicity. The U.S. Food and Drug Administration (FDA) doesn't have any limitations on food residues, and the Cornucopia Institute found residues from hexane in soybean oil in 2009.[52]

Another study[53] reported that five solvents were actually used in the production of cotton seed oil, which are hexane, benzene, acetone, ethyl-ether, and Butanone.

The oil is heated again at temperatures up to 188 degrees Fahrenheit and mixed with acid, sodium hydroxide or sodium carbonate.[54] The oil is then bleached, deodorized and packaged to be sold.

Eating PUFAs Will Decrease Your Lifespan

Despite so much confusion around the PUFA propaganda regarding "heart health," scientists can't deny the reality around PUFA lowering lifespan in mammals.

For example, in the opening paragraphs of a 2006 study published in the journal Aging Cell, entitled "Polyunsaturated fatty acids impair lifespan but have no role for metabolism," the authors are quoted as saying,

"Although generally considered as beneficial components of dietary fats, polyunsaturated fatty acids (PUFA) have been suspected to compromise maximum lifespan in mammals. Specifically, high amounts of phospholipid PUFAs are thought to impair lifespan due to an increase in the susceptibility of membranes to lipid peroxidation and its damaging effect on cellular molecules."[55]

Being "generally considered" as healthy doesn't seem to bode well for PUFAs against the hard facts, specifically that the oxidation of rancid PUFAs in the body damages our cells, causing rapid aging and shorter lifespans.

Scientists have also discovered, time and again,[56] that double bond content in fatty acids is consistently negatively correlated with lifespan in mammals. The more double bond fatty acids, like PUFAs, in the diet, the shorter the lifespan.

To make things worse, PUFAs – along with drugs like statins

that are designed to allegedly try to treat cardiovascular disease - have both been found to cause premature death in studies on hypertensive and diabetic mammals.[57]

In fact, there is literally a heart disease drug called Etomoxir[58] designed to treat heart failure by switching the heart's energy supply from fatty acids over to pyruvate, a product of glucose metabolism, which is more easily converted to energy by the mitochondria. Heart failure is characterized by a fatty acid metabolism, and this is so well-known that a drug that saves people from heart failure has been designed to switch the energy supply back to glucose.

It is absolutely insane that the very things the American Heart Association is recommending to people with cardiovascular disease are actually lowering their chances of living. The scientists researching this subject claim that the reason for statins and vegetable oils causing premature death in diabetic mammals is due to their inhibition of the Vitamin K2-dependent processes in the body, which can also lead to symptoms such as kidney failure, mental disorders, hemorrhaging, and increased tendency for bone fractures.

Fish oil is another culprit in shortening lifespans. Research published in 2002 in the journal Diabetes, Nutrition, and Metabolism found that mammals fed on a high fish oil diet had an uncharacteristically high rate of premature deaths over the study.[59] To quote the authors,

"Deaths were found especially in the fish oil diet group. Compared to the other diet groups, plasma insulin levels of the fish oil diet group were significantly increased 3 months after the start of the diet and remained higher for another 3 months."

In a cohort from the Sydney Heart Study in Australia,[60] a large set of data of 458 men with a history of cardiovascular disease was analyzed. The results were disturbing to say the least, but completely in line with everything we've been discussing here about the dangers of PUFA.

The researchers were analyzing data in order to determine the effectiveness of switching from saturated fats in the diet, such as butter, to PUFA, such as safflower oil, on improving heart health in the men, since this is - after all - the exact recommendation that worldwide medical associations are giving the general public.

The results were the exact opposite of what the "heart healthy guidelines" would have you believe. In the words of the researchers,

"Advice to substitute polyunsaturated fats for saturated fats is a key component of worldwide dietary guidelines for coronary heart disease risk reduction. In this cohort, substituting dietary linoleic acid in place of saturated fats increased the rates of death from all causes, coronary heart disease, and cardiovascular disease. An updated meta-analysis of linoleic acid intervention trials showed no evidence of cardiovascular benefit. These findings could have important implications for worldwide dietary advice to substitute omega 6 linoleic acid, or polyunsaturated fats in general, for saturated fats."

And unsurprisingly, these findings never hit the news and remain hidden in the annals of publicly funded research databases.

Eating PUFA Lowers Your Sexual Hormones and Hurts Your Reproductive Capacity

This is one of my all-time favorite topics to write about: sex hormones.

I've written an entire 580 page book on the subject, called Master Your T, all about how to naturally increase your testosterone levels by using smart nutrition, supplementation, training, lifestyle factors, and by correcting key micronutrient deficiencies. So if you're interested in the subject in far more detail, I highly recommend reading that.

It was during my journey overcoming my own low testosterone, bringing it up from 11 ng/dL to 1192 ng/dL that I stumbled across a study that first introduced me to the idea that PUFAs are severely damaging to your sexual health.

The study[61] is titled, "Testosterone and cortisol in relationship to dietary nutrients and resistance exercise," and it was originally published in the Journal of Applied Physiology.

This study is great for many reasons, demonstrating key relationships between steroid hormones and diet elements such as different types of fats, carbohydrates, and protein consumption in active men, but the big thing that stuck out to me first was quite literally a dose dependent lowering of testosterone when consuming PUFAs.

The researchers highlighted the need to have a higher ratio of Saturated Fat to PUFA in the diet in order to reach higher testosterone levels. This once again, corroborates the idea we've been learning all along - that saturated fat is a far preferable fat source over PUFAs for anyone who wants to be hormonally and metabolically healthy.

In women, PUFA consumption is linked to increased estrogen levels and decreased progesterone during pregnancy,[62] which is potentially very dangerous to the health of the mother and baby, as progesterone is the key protective hormone that women need to optimize.

Progesterone is supposed to be naturally high during pregnancy, which is why most pregnant women are beaming with glowing skin and amazing hair.

Another interesting study called The Israeli Paradox[63] pointed out the seeming "paradox" that despite widespread recommendations of eating a high PUFA diet for "heart health," Israelis - who nationally have one of the highest PUFA concentrated diets of any country - also have staggeringly high incidence of cardiovascular disease, diabetes, obesity and hypertension.

Vegetarians, who consumed higher levels of PUFAs due to self-imposed dietary restrictions, have been found in the research to have higher levels of SHBG - sex hormone binding globulin - a protein whose sole purpose is to bind steroid hormones like testosterone, rendering them unable to be used by the body on receptor sites.[64] This is not good.

And to make the case worse for fish oil supplements, human subjects who consume fish oil have been found to have up to 50% higher cortisol levels[65] than non-fish oil consumers. Cortisol is the body's chief stress hormone, and acts antithetically to important sex hormones like testosterone and progesterone.

Eating PUFAs Will Damage Your Thyroid

Out of all the glands in the body, the two you should pay utmost attention to optimizing naturally are your pituitary and your thyroid.

The thyroid is intricately tied throughout the body's endocrine system feedback loops, so any malfunction in the gland will have wide reaching consequences.

The thyroid is also the chief regulator of your metabolism, so -

bringing this back to Thermo principles - it is very important for regulating the flow of energy throughout your body, from the cellular level up to the tissues, organs, organ systems, and the entire organism.

The thyroid regulates metabolism mainly through the action of the thyroid hormones T3 (triiodothyronine) and T4 (thyroxine), which are secreted and interact with many different tissues in the body with varying levels of sensitivity to the hormones.

PUFA, unsurprisingly at this point, also damages your thyroid gland.

While certain vegetables and goitrogen containing foods such as legumes should be avoided due to their ability to block iodine uptake in the thyroid, causing hormonal production problems, PUFAs specifically act on harming your T3 thyroid hormone activity in multiple ways.

Research has shown us[66] that PUFA suppresses thyroid signaling, suppressing these thyroid hormone levels and causing weight gain in humans and other mammals. By inhibiting the thyroid function, PUFAs slow down your metabolism.

Researchers have also found that even on lower calorie diets, people who consumed PUFAs were able to gain body fat despite being in a calorie deficit.[67]

One really cool study found that the ingestion of PUFA directly inhibited specific enzymes that break down fat tissue.[68] The more PUFAs were consumed, the less the body could break down body fat. This type of finding perfectly explains why people who have hypothyroid issues also have a lot of trouble losing body fat in general.

Not only is the PUFA damaging your metabolic functioning and thyroid hormone production and signaling, but it is also blocking the very enzymes that are responsible for breaking down fat tissue.

Hopefully this is all starting to make sense to you and help you get some clarity on what may be a major "sneaky" source of your health issues.

So here's the elephant in the room...

So the question I keep mulling over is this...

Why in the fuck is PUFA still in our food supply? And why isn't anybody educating people about the dangers of consuming all of the vegetable oils, seed oils, nut oils, fish oils, and frankenstein cooking oils?

We've funded mountains of public research with our tax dollars that demonstrates time and time again just how massively dangerous PUFAs are for human consumption.

Yet nobody is talking about it.

Nobody is taking action on getting PUFAs out of our food supply.

I think that needs to change. And I for one, am ready to help.

The first step for all of us is on the personal level. As consumers, we "vote" with the money we spend at grocery stores and restaurants.

When consumers start movements in a direction, and continue to vote with their dollars by picking better options, restaurants and stores have no choice but to respond by offering better and better options, because they risk losing business if they don't accommodate their customers.

Also, we need to make sure we keep ourselves healthy and our families and friends healthy. I would urge you to audit your kitchen pantry, and choose better places to eat out that don't use vegetable oils for cooking.

Don't let your children consume PUFAs because the oils can be especially toxic to a growing developing body.

Ask your local restaurants if they can cook your food for you in butter or coconut oil instead of their cooking oils. Many of them will be happy to do it for you.

Now that you're aware of the huge health risks associated with consuming excess PUFAs, it's your responsibility to bring this awareness to others and take action in your life to turn your health around.

If enough of us start demanding better options from our favorite restaurants, the world will start to change for the better of our public health.

CHAPTER FIVE

EAT LESS PROTEIN

THE LAW OF AMINO ACID BALANCE

The idea of eating less protein goes completely against everything we hear in the media or read in dieting or fitness magazines. "Eat more protein" is such a common piece of nutrition advice that it may seem completely ludicrous to advise otherwise. However, it's important for you to understand that not all amino acids are created equal. Amino acids are the subunits that make up proteins, and as micronutrients, they are built with different structural makeup, and have far-reaching effects on the body as a whole - sometimes positive, sometimes negative. Great health requires a specific balance of amino acids within the body that is becoming increasingly less common in our modern food culture. Muscle meats, which are the most common modern protein sources for the majority of the population, are composed of specific amino acids that, when consumed in excess and without the presence of the right protective amino acids found in other parts of the animal that are no longer eaten often in our diets, can be detrimental to your health.

Open any microbiology textbook and you will read that "proteins are the building blocks of life."[1]

And it's true. Proteins are the most common molecules in the cell, more common than lipids, carbohydrates and all other molecules combined.

A protein is made up of chains of amino acid subunits.[2]

They're used for a staggering amount of different functions within the human body, from movement, to structural support, storage, cellular communication, digestion, and more.

For the sake of this book, I want to highlight the fact that the amino acids that make up a protein are vitally important to the structural integrity of that protein, and not all amino acids are created equal. Some of them have a more protective, and positive effect on the human body, while others have negative effects in high quantities.

Overall protein itself as a macronutrient is a more widely known way of referring to protein, so we're also going to treat it as such, looking at a few things in this section namely how much protein does the human body really need to consume from food and what are the best food sources to get it from with the most favorable amino acid profiles.

Protective Amino Acids

The amino acids that make up a protein can have a wide range of different effects on the body, often acting to exert hormone-like functions. This becomes an important reality to pay attention to because in times of stress, for example when glycogen has been depleted, the body will convert tissue into free amino acids in order to produce more glucose.

Some of these free amino acids released during stress periods, namely tryptophan and cysteine, can suppress thyroid gland function, and in high enough quantities can be toxic.

These are what I refer to as "Destructive Amino Acids."

There are also "Protective Amino Acids" such as glycine, proline, taurine, and arginine, that when in the free state can exert very positive effects on important body functions by protecting important endocrine functions, such as the activities of the thyroid gland, while also aiding in shutting down the stress response.

To be clear, an amino acid isn't positive or negative due to its state of 'being' or as some sort of inherent property, however the dose makes the poison, so I like to classify them as Protective or Destructive as a simple way to consider the potential effect of having large amounts of that amino acid present in the body at any moment.

This type of thinking is helpful when we're making our choices about potential protein sources that we get from our food.

With protective amino acids, glycine is king. The positive effects of consuming more glycine are far reaching in the body.

Due to cultural shifts, glycine intake from the forms of collagen and animal gelatin has drastically dropped as most people no longer eat "whole animal" or consume bone broth, joints, ligaments and so forth. These are all extremely rich sources of glycine.

Glycine is essential for the production of bile acid, creatine, nucleic acids, and porphyrins, supporting many important processes within the nervous system and the gut.[3]

Glycine is neuroprotective[4] and can lower oxidative stress[5] and it has been shown in the research to help improve all sleep parameters in humans.[6] Supplementation with glycine has also been shown to get rid of fatigue caused by sleep deprivation.[7]

Glycine mixed with niacin and glutamine was demonstrated to give men a 70% boost in natural growth hormone production in just 3 weeks![8] This is likely due to the fact that glycine is one of the main stimulatory agents for the pituitary gland[9] to naturally secrete more hGH.[10]

It doesn't just help growth, but glycine supplementation has also been shown to increase the metabolic rate and food efficiency in mammals.[11]

Glycine supplementation has also been shown to support the healing of the liver by protecting it against cellular damage[12] and removing excess lipid accumulation in the liver (fatty liver).[13]

Proline is another key protective amino acid.

Proline supplementation contributes to increased natural collagen production,[14] which leads to improved skin quality. Similar to glycine, proline contributes to boosting growth parameters in animals as well.[15]

Another beneficial amino acid is alanine. Alanine helps your body properly convert glucose into energy and aids the liver in its natural detoxification processes.[16] It is also known for increasing immune function while providing energy to the brain and central nervous system and stimulating muscle growth.

Arginine also has positive effects on muscle growth,[17] as well as helping erectile dysfunction, strengthening the immune system, improving insulin sensitivity, improving spermatogenesis, and increasing blood flow.[18]

Destructive Amino Acids

On the flip side, certain specific amino acids have been shown to be destructive in their influence in excess. I point these out, because excess is common with these three amino acids due to the high amount of them present in the typical modern diet: methionine, cysteine, and tryptophan.

First off, all three of them have been shown in research to inhibit healthy thyroid function.[19]

Tryptophan causes an increase in central nervous system fatigue,[20] increases oxidative stress in the brain,[21] and wildly enough excess tryptophan has been correlated with white[22] and grey hair[23] in humans, likely due to an interplay with creating a copper deficiency.

Due to its sedative effects, tryptophan impairs measured reaction time and psychomotor skills in humans.[24]

Cysteine has been shown to act as an excitotoxin, causing brain damage.[25]

It's also been shown to reduce glutathione levels in the brain,[26] damaging brain cell membranes in the process. Cysteine's capacity for neurotoxicity has been studied quite extensively in the medical literature.[27]

Cysteine's negative effects aren't just limited to the brain and thyroid gland, but it can also damage the kidneys.[28]

Dietary methionine is another nasty one, having been demonstrated to cause intestinal cancers as well.[29]

Restricting methionine helps to improve thyroid functioning.[30]

The Truth About Protein Supplements

Protein is a big market.

Globally, consumers spent $14 billion on protein supplements in 2018,[31] most of it marketed for muscle building purposes.

But there is a major problem... most of the supplements were found to be contaminated with dangerous compounds like heavy metals lead (70% of products) and cadmium (74% of products)[32] and even arsenic.[33]

At first glance, it may seem like the worst offenders would be the cheapest brands, such as protein powders you'd find in Walmart or at the bottom of the bargain bin, however the testing has shown that in fact many of the brands that people see as "premium" brands, charging 2-4x as much on retail pricing over the cheap brands, are the most contaminated with mercury, cadmium, lead, and BPA: brands like Sun Warrior, Vega, and Garden of Life.

Most of the contaminated protein powders are whey, but plant based proteins were also surveyed and contained high levels of the same dangerous compounds as well.

One of the main problems with proteins like whey, is the way it needs to be processed, and the lack of quality control around original sourcing for the dairy itself.

As we know, the source of your food matters, so things become problematic when cheap estrogen-laden dairy is used to produce the average whey protein that you can buy in supplement powders.

Whey is called a complete protein since it contains the full range of 9 "essential" amino acids[35] needed to be classified as such. However the term "complete protein" isn't much more than a marketing gimmick used to get consumers to believe that whey is somehow superior to other forms of protein. There is nothing desirable about adding more tryptophan and methionine to your diet.

Whey is hailed as great for muscle building, weight loss, and overall general wellness however the science itself does not back up even these basic claims... aside from the fact that most whey is highly contaminated with the aforementioned heavy metals and endocrine disrupting chemicals.

With respect to muscle building, whey protein consumption has actually been shown in research to lower important anabolic hormones like testosterone and growth hormone[36-38] while simultaneously increasing estrogen levels.[39-41]

Mountains of research have looked directly at muscle gaining protocols using whey protein and have found no positive effect.[42-48]

Whey consumption is also directly linked to acne in humans, especially young men.[49-53]

Usually touted for weight loss and appetite control, the studies demonstrate that whey protein actually does the opposite, causing no decrease in appetite or food intake regulation.[54-57]

While increasing insulin resistance... which, taken together is a recipe for weight gain.[58-61]

Plant-based proteins aren't much better. Aside from contaminants as well, plant based proteins offer another obstacle: protease inhibitors.

Protease inhibitors are a natural defense mechanism of the plant.[62]

How Much Protein Do You Really Need?

Proteins are broken down into the individual amino acids during digestion and then reassimilated in the body to form the different proteins that our body needs at that time. These can be anything from tissues that are needed to be formed in the body to enzymes that are needed to speed up reactions happening throughout the body. This is necessary for proper metabolic functioning, movement, and structure of the human body.[63-64]

So needless to say protein is a necessity on the human diet, but what is the optimal amount of protein, how much do we really need, are we getting too much?

Many people believe that if you are training then you need at the very least 1 gram of protein per pound of body weight, but this simply is not the case. The more that I dive into the research of protein the more I realize we don't need as much as we have been led to believe.

There are two ways that protein is measured in research, either grams per kilogram, or grams per pound of body weight. I prefer to speak in terms of grams per pound of body weight.

It has been shown in several places that one of if not the greatest bodybuilder of all time mr Arnold Schwarzenneger only ate about .7 grams of protein per pound of body weight and about 60% of his diet coming from carbs.[65]

The research says that he was right in the sweet spot.

With the minimum effective dose of protein ideally being .5 grams per pound of bodyweight. The maximum effective dose has been shown to be .82 grams of protein per pound of bodyweight, with anything over this amount showing no beneficial effect, actually in many cases causing more harm than good.

Due to the excess ammonia and heavy work that protein puts on the kidneys you are really just looking to develop early dependence on dialysis when you chronically eat more protein than this.

So how do you know what end of the spectrum you need to be on?

For younger people you can easily get by on the lower end of the spectrum with no ill side effects coming from muscle loss, or associated disorders. As for people on the older side of human chronological age it would be better to try and stick to the higher end of the spectrum in order to ensure that some form of muscle wasting like sarcopenia doesn't catch up with you.[66-69]

It has also been shown that a lower protein intake (like the intake within the range that I have been talking about) is associated with a longer life. Excess protein has been associated with lowered NAD+ levels and thus a shorter lifespan due to the effects of mitochondria and telomere shortening.[70-71]

CHAPTER SIX

DON'T EAT VEGETABLES

THE LAW OF PLANT DEFENSE

Vegetables, defined as the leaves and stems of plants, have evolved highly sophisticated natural pesticides and toxin mechanisms specifically to discourage insects and animals from eating them. The chief function of leaves on a plant is to facilitate photosynthesis by absorbing light energy from the sun and carbon dioxide into the stomata from the surrounding atmosphere, which allow the plant to grow and trigger cellular respiration, and it therefore makes perfect sense that a process so vital to the survival of the plant should be protected. Since the metabolic functioning of an animal is the key to its long term health, it is not surprising that plant defense chemicals would have specific anti-metabolic effects on animals, in order to provide a negative evolutionary stimulus, allowing the plant to protect its most vital components, its leaves and stem, from becoming a routine part of an animal's diet. Focus your dietary habits, rather, around consuming the fruits and roots of plants, since they are nutrient-dense, do not contain anti-metabolic toxin defenses, and are rich in metabolism-stoking carbohydrates.

Plants are fascinating to study.

When a plant is injured, it naturally secretes an increased amount of toxins, in order to protect itself from the predator, and to discourage being consumed.

Plant toxins, released from the leaves, have been found to have specifically negative effects on animal tissues, which is quite amazing to think about. For example, a certain phytotoxin from the plant may be able to block enzyme action in an animal's body, sometimes inflicting significant damage, but when another plant is exposed to that same phytotoxin, its analogous enzymatic functioning stays intact, unaffected.

Plants are very powerful, and must be respected as such.

Extracts from leaves can prove to be extremely useful, especially in natural medicine applications. However, eating the leaves of the plant as vegetables is not advised for health reasons.

Vegetables are not necessary.

In high amounts, raw vegetables are potentially harmful to your health, inhibiting important enzymes, leaching nutrients from the body, and negatively impacting the thyroid gland as well, since many of them are rich in goitrogens, which block iodine uptake in the thyroid, hurting your ability to properly produce thyroid hormones.

Vegetables are also rich in anti-metabolic toxins such as phenols, tannins, trypsin-inhibitors, and agglutinins, among other things.

On the other hand, a fully ripened fruit contains no toxins, which makes sense because it must be eaten, so its indigestible seeds can be transported, fertilized, and redistributed to another place in the Earth where the plant can grow anew.

Roots, or tubers, are also nutrient-rich and protected from grazing predators underground, so they never developed anti-digestive anti-metabolic defense toxins like the leaves. In fact, the roots contain pro-digestive prebiotic fibers that are favorable for supporting the human gut microbiome.

What is A Vegetable?

The working definition of what constitutes a vegetable has actually been strangely controversial.

However, for the purposes of this book I am going to define the plants that we'll be discussing: fruits, vegetables, and tubers - in the following, most widely agreed-upon way:

1. A vegetable constitutes the stems and leaves, for example celery and broccoli (stems) and kale, spinach, lettuce (leaves)
2. A fruit contains seeds, and is the structure that develops from the ovaries of a flowering plant: for example,

apples, peaches, grapes, mangoes etc. One common misconception is that fruits are only sweet. There are actually plenty of savory fruits, for example eggplant, tomatoes, zucchini, avocados, olives, squash, and bell peppers.

3. Tubers are roots. They're so dense in nutrients that they literally sprout and sustain their own plants if left unharvested. Potatoes, sweet potatoes, carrots, turnips, and beets all fall under this category.

As you can see, most of what the average person would consider a vegetable, is actually NOT a vegetable. And all of the ones that most people would actually agree tasted any good, are not vegetables... They are fruits and tubers.

One thing that struck me as interesting is to just take a step back and simply examine the facts about the differences between how fruits, vegetables, and tubers grow. And what this might tell us about their specific value or purpose in their evolutionary role with humans.

It would appear after a basic examination of the facts, that fruits are meant to be eaten.

First off, they're jam packed with nutrients, and if someone was to eat even a small range of different fruits regularly, they would fulfill most if not all of their dietary micronutrient needs.

Another thing that is interesting is the fast ripening cycles of fruits. They go through fast growing and ripening cycles, and all contain seeds (most of the seeds/pits are hard and inedible) that regrow the trees/bushes/vines after consumption, even if the human/animal just drops it on the ground haphazardly. This is a really convincing and genius pollination technique that ensures their long term survival but also their relationship with animals/ people that will eat them and spread their seed for them after.

Vegetables on the other hand are not this way, they require more careful cultivation and release small amounts of bitter toxins as a defense mechanism against being eaten by animals/insects... quite the opposite of fruits.

Vegetables have developed these defense systems specifically to NOT be eaten by insects or other animals. While the leaves and stems of certain plants do contain nutrients, they're not necessarily the best sources of those nutrients for humans to consume.

They contain almost zero calories, which evolutionarily speaking is a downside, and the human stomach doesn't have much of a capacity for massive leaf or stem consumption due to the high load of cellulose and fiber, whereas other species of mammals have developed stomach systems, like that of grazing cows, that are meant to be able to handle massive all-day-long consumption of these grasses, stems, and leaves.

It simply does not make any evolutionary sense for a human to NEED to consume the leaves or stems of certain plants in order to be healthy.

The low caloric density coupled with high fiber and non-exclusive nutrients all point to a reasonable conclusion that humans do not need to consume vegetables - they are likely, in fact, more of a luxury in today's modern world, but most definitely not necessary.

Now let's consider tubers.

Tubers are literally roots that are so nutritious they will sprout their own plants, and feed those plants with their nutrients. They also gather nutrients from the soil around them. Hell, you don't even have to plant a tuber in the ground for it to grow... if you leave a potato out on the kitchen counter, for example, it will sprout without water or outside nutrition. Tubers also have a generally very appealing taste to humans and other animals. The starchy carbohydrates are easily digested and also contain prebiotic fiber which is great for human intestinal flora.

A lot of people hate the taste of vegetables, yet they carry around some kind of ridiculous guilt about not eating them regularly. This guilt isn't necessary. You can be extremely healthy by getting your nutrients from fruits and tubers and you'll live to a ripe old age without ever eating another bitter leaf of kale again.

Kale, by the way, is merely a modern cultural nutrition fad. It's not fit for human consumption, yet people have been swindled into thinking it's healthy.

In fact, the kale fad has done more harm than good, and in such an underhanded way that most people won't even realize it's the kale that is giving them issues.

Why?

Well let's examine some facts about kale...

Kale was originally grown with the intention of feeding sheep since it is so inexpensive to grow. Farmers were feeding kale to their sheep as an alternate food source, yet they started to realize that lambs were being born with goiter, or basically a swollen and poorly functioning thyroid gland.

Researchers experimented with kale on sheep and rabbits with disturbing results. Turns out kale does contain a goitrogen, thiocyanate, which is chemically very similar to deadly cyanide. Some young lambs were stillborn, their brain development stunted by their goiters. The consumption of kale had blocked their thyroid's ability to function properly even in the presence of proper iodine consumption.

With many modern people consuming little iodine, it's no wonder the instances of hypothyroidism are rising every year. Meanwhile, kale is being turned into every type of junk food imaginable, from PUFA fried kale chips to kale shakes, this anti-thyroid leafy vegetable is going to do some real damage if not exposed.

Scientists, when they first started studying kale, never considered that humans would someday consider kale a "health food." Back then it was only food for livestock. But even though people weren't noshing on kale chips all day, kale managed to poison them. Cows grazing on kale transferred its poisons to their milk,[1] affecting the thyroid development of children who drank it and causing an epidemic of goiter in Tasmania.[2]

Kale is also rich in sulfur and compounds that convert to sulfur, which is the chemical that makes rotten eggs smell putrid. One metabolite of sulfur, S-methyl cysteine sulphoxide, is known to cause "kale poisoning" – severe hemolytic anemia, a life-threatening breakdown of red blood cells, in livestock.[3] Poor sulfur digestion is associated with many[4] serious illnesses in humans,[5] though whether it causes them or merely exacerbates them remains to be seen.[6]

It makes sense that Kale would be dangerous given it evolved in an evolutionary war against those that dare to eat its leaves from aurochs to insects.

My point in using kale as an example isn't to scare anybody, it's merely to point out that the evolutionary role of leaves is not as benign as you may have first considered. Since leaves are constantly exposed to potential predators, the plants develop very effective chemical defense mechanisms against being eaten.

Wouldn't it make more sense to eat something nutritious that will actually make you healthier and needs you to eat it, like fruit?

Fiber Myth

One of the most common arguments people use for recommending that you eat vegetables is the fact that vegetables are a rich, consistent source of dietary fiber. And like all conventional health wisdom, the fiber myth is fascinating when you actually dig into the science behind it.

Ask anyone what they think about fiber and they'll tell you "you should eat more fiber" and "fiber is healthy for you." The general consensus among the population is that "more is better" when it comes to fiber consumption.

As you can probably tell, based on where I am leading this... It's not that simple.

This idea has become conventional wisdom thanks to wide scale marketing campaigns, mostly from General Mills, in order to sell high fiber cereals to consumers. A lot of the marketing centers around heart health, weight loss (if you're full, you can't eat more, right?), or some sort of "doctor recommendation" about daily fiber intake.

All of it is very misleading, so I want to clear the air by taking a good look at actual scientific research around the subject, and putting that up against whether or not consuming more fiber is actually healthy according to our Thermo definition of health regarding micronutrient deficiencies and hormonal balance.

Fiber originally was thought to be dose dependent in the effects that it had in the human body.

This theory came from the thought that fruits and vegetables which are usually high in fiber help prevent things like obesity, diabetes, heart disease, and other chronic conditions.[7-10] What they didn't think about was the decrease in calories and most likely body weight that accompanied this.

Studies have been conducted where they supplement fiber on its own in an unchanged diet and no protective benefits have been shown.

But nevertheless dogma has its way and the common idea of the dose dependent manner has made its way through the years. Fiber is necessary in order for optimal health, but too much can be a bad thing especially when it is in an isolated form such as when it is added to cereals and other fiber fortified foods, or when it comes from raw vegetables in their naturally indigestible forms.

Too much fiber has been shown to be harmful to the bacteria in your gut and cause several chronic digestive issues such as diverticulitis. High fiber diets also have no beneficial effects in weight loss and satiety,[11-13] it doesn't help with the prevention of colon cancer,[14-18] and can actually worsen a lot of gut related issues.[19-22]

There are a few different types of fiber. The two simplest categories are soluble and insoluble fiber.[23-24] Soluble fiber attracts water and turns to gel when it goes through the digestive system, which slows down the digestion process. Soluble fiber is found in oat bran, barley, nuts, seeds, beans, lentils, peas, and some fruits and vegetables. It is also found in psyllium, a common fiber supplement.

Insoluble fiber is found in foods such as wheat bran, vegetables, and whole grains. It adds bulk to the stool and appears to help food pass more quickly through the stomach and intestines.

Forms of soluble fiber such as oligofructose and inulin, both from fruits, help to maintain the beneficial bacteria in the intestines by feeding them (being a prebiotic fiber). When you feed the bacteria in your gut they are able to better absorb nutrients; ramping up the energy flow throughout the body.

Human breast milk prebiotics have a substantial impact on the growth of beneficial bacteria in the gut. It is made by the mother to allow for the proper growth of bacteria to accumulate in the gut of the baby.

Can we have too much of a good thing though?

We can see that Asian men on a typical Asian diet that is higher in fiber is relative to the low amount of testosterone that accompanies Asian men.[25-27] A diet too high in fiber can have a negative effect on protective hormones such as testosterone and other androgens in men.[28-35] It increases SHBG which is the molecule that binds to the androgens and renders them inactive so they can't attach to the receptor, and they can't serve their purpose.

But this effect isn't just seen in men, it is also seen in women.[36]

On top of the negative effects that it can have on the hormonal balance in the human body it can also cause a significant increase in the amount of gas that you produce.[37]

However most of the negative effects are seen with insoluble fiber, the type of fiber that just passes through the system aka the type of fiber that is seen in vegetables, cereal grains, and other types of processed foods.

Foods that are high in insoluble are also high in things like phytic acid and can cause malabsorption. Chronically this will lead to nutrient deficiencies.[38] When fiber is in excess in the body specifically in the insoluble form it can inhibit the absorption of macronutrients, yes MACROnutrients.[39-40]

Resistant starch is the beneficial insoluble fiber that can be found in things like psyllium, carrots, and cold cooked potatoes.[41] It helps with insulin sensitivity and secretion,[42-43] and has been shown to help improve metabolism and liver function through downregulating liver related inflammation.[44]

However soluble fiber which is found in whole foods and

typically in the most Thermo approved foods is very good in the right amounts. Soluble fiber is very beneficial in down regulation of estrogen receptors which is correlated with decreased risk of breast cancer.[45]

Beneficial soluble fiber such as oligofructose the soluble fiber that comes from fruits is the most beneficial. Showing an increase in satiety hormones,[46] a decrease in ghrelin which is the hormone that tells the body that it is hungry, protects the liver from damage,[47] enhances bone mineralization,[48] preventing mucosal inflammatory disorders,[49] and prevention and treatment of disease.[50]

Oligofructose has also been shown to have the best physiological benefits out of several different types of fibers.[51] Studies have also shown that these prebiotics are very beneficial in the early stages of development to lower instances of allergies and infections.[52] Although this is the most beneficial type of fiber the benefits start to falter off whenever consumption goes over 25 grams per day.[53]

This does not mean if you are getting 35-40 grams of fiber a day you should completely change your food intake.

If you enjoy Thermo Diet approved food sources such as fruits and tubers, you'll naturally get the proper ratios and amount of soluble fiber you need on a daily basis to be in vibrant health.

However do not go out of your way to get extreme amounts of

fiber. It is completely useless and can even be harmful. If you are over 45 grams of fiber daily I would make sure to really pay attention to your body. If your digestion begins to falter then you might want to take a look at the amount of fiber you are consuming, from vegetables or other sources.

CHAPTER SEVEN

BALANCE YOUR HORMONES

THE LAW OF LEVERAGE

Your body is only healthy when your hormones are balanced. Hormones are the key to not just restoring your health to the Thermo State, but also to maintaining it and improving it over time. Your endocrine system is a complex framework of feedback loops - natural compensation mechanisms - with hormones either supporting or suppressing one another. When your stress hormones are chronically high, your protective hormones are low, and vice versa. While hormones might seem complex, they are in fact quite simple to manipulate; you manipulate them right now all the time, without even knowing it. All day long, with every decision you make, you're constantly either supporting your protective hormones or your stress hormones. It's time to become aware of which habits and actions you take are either helping you, or hurting you.

In your mind's eye, picture a rock stuck in a funnel.

Now envision trying to pour some water into the top of that funnel. With very little water able to get around the crevices of that rock, the water starts building up to the top of the funnel, eventually overflowing.

If you dump the water out, then try a different liquid, or maybe something else, like a powder, the same thing will happen. Little, if any, will get through the funnel. It's all being blocked.

That's what my brain tumor was doing to me ten years ago, only it was acting like this rock in a funnel inside my pituitary gland: the control center for my endocrine system.

The pituitary communicates with, and receives feedback from vital organs like your thyroid gland, adrenals, liver, and reproductive organs.

When it's not functioning properly, like in my case, everything starts to go horribly wrong. None of these important organs - your thyroid, liver, reproductive organs, or adrenals - can get the signaling and feedback they need in order to keep your body healthy.

When I finally found the tumor on an MRI, I started rifling through my textbooks to find any information I could on how to help myself get out of this mess without using surgery or drugs. Cracking open *Williams Textbook of Endocrinology*, it became evident that my problem wasn't only about the hypothalamus not being able to get the right input through my pituitary out to the body, but none of these other glands could send the right feedback back through the pituitary properly either!

I quickly realized that the endocrine system functions entirely on feedback loops; hormone signaling is cyclical, not linear. Nearly every medical illustration in the textbook has cyclical arrows drawn out, demonstrating these feedback loops between every major gland in the body, and the pituitary is right in the middle of it all.

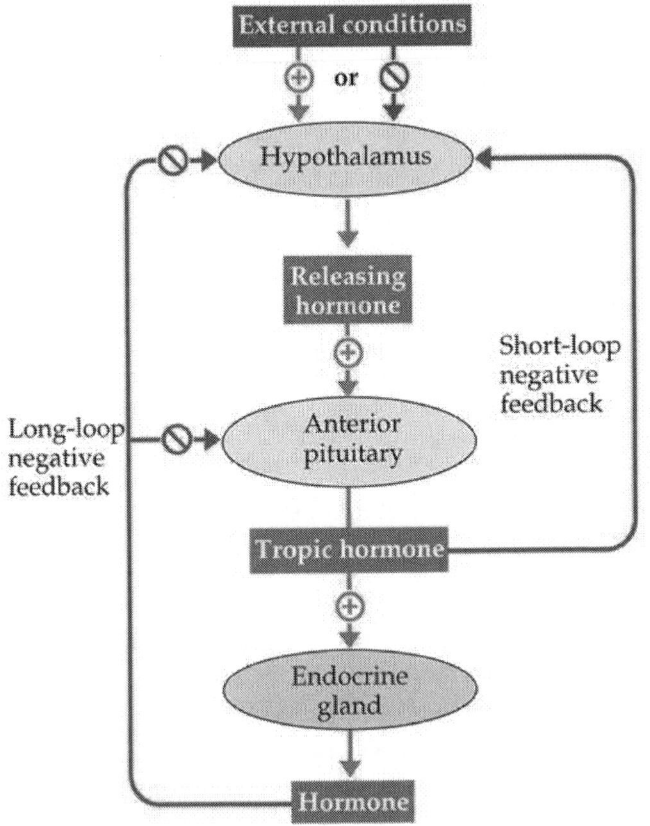

Before that point, I had very little understanding that the body was so systemically integrated. It's just one big system, and all the glands inside of it communicate with one another. And they do so, with hormones. These hormone loops help the glands regulate one another, to stay in a state of balance.

All of my doctors were "specialists," only viewing the body through one lens: *their specialty.* They seemed to all think of the body as a compartmentalized jigsaw puzzle, focusing on just one area without any sense of what the big picture really was.

It reminded me a lot of the ancient parable of the three blind men and the elephant, the Indian story about three blind men coming upon an elephant. They all touch different parts of the elephant and describe what it is to one another. Having different opinions that they're convinced are the truth, they start to fight with one another over which one is telling the truth. None of them can see the big picture - the whole elephant.

Once I understood that the body is just one whole system, and that hormone feedback loops were the key to restoring my health naturally, everything changed. I felt empowered. I knew that, if I could just figure out how to signal enough of the right positive feedback from my body back into my brain, while eliminating things that caused negative feedback, that I might just be able to override that damned "rock" in my funnel to get things working properly again.

And it took a lot of effort, research, lifestyle changes, and consistency, *but I did just that.*

What Are Hormones?

The easiest way to think about hormones, is to see them as chemical messengers. Think of a paper boy, riding around the neighborhood on his bicycle, bringing newspapers to everyone's house.

Endocrine hormones are like the bicycle-riding paperboy, riding along the bloodstream to deliver the message they were sent for, by entering the "front door" of a receptor site on the surface of a target cell.

Paracrine hormones are similar, but they stay closer to home, more like if you were walking over to your next-door neighbor's house to give them a tray of cookies as a Christmas gift.

Some hormones have a long-distance job to accomplish, and others stay local, usually just signaling to adjacent cells.

Now here's the really cool thing... picture yourself going online to a shopping website like Amazon. Maybe you need to order some cleaning supplies regularly to clean your home, so you pay to "subscribe" to some different sprays, soaps, and paper towels to be delivered to your house every month. Amazon processes the order, packages the products in their warehouse, and sends out a delivery van to bring them to your house, possibly over hundreds of miles.

A few months from now, you realize that you overestimated how many cleaning supplies you needed, so now you have a surplus... enough soap stockpiled in your storage closet to last you another few months. You don't need to reorder any more for a while.

Now you go back to Amazon and "pause" your subscription.

You just participated in a tangible feedback loop. By starting a subscription, you told Amazon that you needed soap. So they produced and delivered the products to you. By later pausing your subscription, you told Amazon to stop sending you so much soap.

Your endocrine organs work the same way! It's really quite simple to understand.

But let's say, a couple months later, you start running out of soap again. You've been cleaning a lot, and now it's time to turn your subscription back on to restock your supplies. You go to Amazon's website, log in to your account, and see a message on the screen saying, "We're sorry, due to manufacturing & supplier problems, we no longer sell cleaning supplies."

Now what? Now you have to go find them somewhere else, maybe drive to the local store. It's way less convenient and more expensive, not to mention it's costing you additional gas money and time out of your day.

To make things worse, when you get to your local store, they don't have all the exact cleaning supplies you need. You'll just have to make-due, you don't want your house to turn into a disgusting cesspit after all. After a few months of this, you make your routine trip to the local store, and walk up to an empty shelf. No cleaning supplies. Everyone else in your town was facing the same problem, so eventually the store ran out of cleaning supplies and the clerk tells you more won't be back in stock for a few weeks.

As you walk out the door, you see a newspaper on the stand with the headline reading, **"Nationwide Soap Shortage: Major Cleaning Chemical Manufacturers Go Bankrupt."**

In this case, your feedback loop was noticeably disturbed: you needed more supplies, but the most convenient, efficient, and affordable supplier could no longer give you what you needed. You had to make an additional effort to find sub-par resources to get the original job done.

Then your sub-par supplier ran out of supplies. You realize this is a much bigger issue than you originally thought - there's a systemic, nationwide shortage of the raw materials needed to make cleaning supplies. Now what are you supposed to do to keep your home clean?

While this is obviously merely a metaphorical demonstration, very similar feedback patterns happen with your hormones inside your body all the time, including issues with production and raw material supply.

To be produced properly, hormones need raw materials. This is why we see rapid drops in some hormones' production when the body is deficient in vitamins, minerals, and amino acids. Or why we see over-production of certain hormones when too much raw material is flooded into the system without the proper regulation from other hormonal feedback, for example in cases of estrogen excess with too much exposure to environmental estrogenics and unbalanced methionine and tryptophan levels.

Another common situation with hormone imbalance occurs when an organ in the feedback loop system is not functioning properly. One easy example is when your liver is overproducing the protein SHBG (sex hormone binding globulin), which can occur for a range of different reasons. With too much SHBG in the blood, your sex hormones, like testosterone, become over-bound, and cannot get through "the front door" of the receptor sites they need to enter.

This would be akin to someone walking up to your front door and stealing the Amazon box full of cleaning supplies off your front porch.

Now that we have a basic grasp on the concept of hormone feedback loops within your endocrine system, let's take a deeper look at the two main classes of hormones you need to start focusing on for proper hormonal balance: *protective hormones* and *stress hormones.*

Protective Hormones: The Angelic Protectors

A fun, and metaphorically interesting, way to think about the differences between the classes of your body's *protective hormones* and *stress hormones*, is to make them analogous to the ancient concept of angels and demons, respectively.

In philosophical considerations of good and evil, it's apparent that one cannot exist without the other. If someone has truly no understanding of what is good, then how can they know what is evil? The definitions of these words, as concepts, rely on one another to be properly understood.

Inside your body, your protective hormones and your stress hormones exist to balance each other out, to run a system of checks-and-balances in order to maintain homeostasis.

This is why measuring isolated hormone levels in blood tests don't give us much in the way of useful data, *until we compare hormone levels against one another.* For example, the T:C ratio (testosterone to cortisol ratio) is one reliable indicator of protective:stress hormone balance that is widely used in research studies, especially with respect to athletic performance, strength, power, endurance, and male reproductive health.

All hormones are needed for your body to be healthy, however, you start to experience serious health issues when the balance is skewed heavily in favor of stress hormones, which happens to be the case for most people in our modern environment.

Physical and psychological stress, alongside unprecedented exposure to environmental estrogenic chemicals, is at an all-time high right now, when compared to any other time in human history. And epidemic level hormonal health issues have been rising rapidly for many decades now, including thyroid dysfunction, sexual dysfunction, hypertension, gut diseases, and many more.

The average person is sadly unaware of the role their hormones are playing in all of their health problems, not to mention they have no way of knowing how to increase their protective hormone production back to a healthy balance in order to keep the rampant over-production of stress hormones in check.

Protective hormones are in low supply, but I'm going to show you how to increase yours naturally.

There are many different hormones constantly working inside your body. They are made in different ways, structurally. Some of them are produced from amino acids, known as *amino acid derived hormones*, such as dopamine, epinephrine, melatonin, norepinephrine, T3, and T4.

Others are referred to as *eicosanoid hormones*, a class of paracrine hormones that signal locally to neighboring cells, and synthesized as a result of PUFA oxidation. Examples are prostaglandins, leukotrienes, prostacyclin, and thromboxane.

Another class, containing a large variety of hormones, is the *peptide hormones,* like LH, FSH, TSH, adiponectin, hCG, GnRH, hGH, leptin, IGF, and many more, which are structurally composed of peptides or proteins molecules.

And finally, we have the *steroid hormones,* many of which you may be familiar with, such as testosterone DHT, estradiol, cortisol, DHEA, progesterone, and aldosterone.

Protective hormones are defined as those that, at naturally high levels, preserve the healthy functioning of vital biological systems needed to thrive, such as sexual reproduction, energy metabolism, regenerative sleep, & executive cognitive functioning.

At healthy production levels, your protective hormones are able to moderate your stress hormones effectively. You feel energetic, relaxed, creative, and sexually charged. You sleep well at night and can maintain a lean physique quite easily.

While there are many protective hormones, the ones we're going to focus on optimizing are:

1. Thyroid hormones T3 and T4
2. Dopamine
3. Testosterone
4. DHT
5. Progesterone
6. LH, FSH, and GnRH

Ultimately, increasing the production of these hormones revolves around taking actions to improve the functioning of three key organs: the pituitary, liver, and thyroid gland.

The most helpful thinking tool I've employed over the years is the concept of thinking in terms of *leverage.* What one thing can I focus on that will get me most of, if not all, the results I'm seeking?

Average people get mediocre results because they don't think this way. Most people will chase too many rabbits at once, only to catch none.

Exceptional people get excellent results by identifying one core focus, then relentlessly pursuing that one thing until they get it. If you pick the right thing to fixate on, it will apply enough leverage to take care of everything else as a byproduct.

And the beautiful thing about leveraged thinking when it comes to protective hormones, is that all of these hormones are involved in the same systems with one another. They communicate to one another constantly. Optimizing them requires doing the same exact things, which I will show you shortly.

Stress Hormones: The Downward Spiral

Like everything in the body, stress hormones serve a specific purpose. For example, cortisol is absolutely needed for survival, rapidly rising in times of acute stress to trigger adrenaline and noradrenaline production to heighten your senses and physical response times in order to avoid getting hit by that speeding taxi as you step off the NYC sidewalk into the street.

Acute, rapid increases in stress hormones aren't necessarily a bad thing. They help you stay alive. Especially when you do something stupid.

Unfortunately, for most of us, our stress hormones aren't just acutely elevated. They're chronically elevated.

The catabolic nature of stress hormones can have a catastrophic negative effect on your health when chronically elevated, quite literally destroying your body in a "slow burn" over decades.

Stress hormones stay chronically elevated because of environmental input into your body, such as prolonged physical or psychological stressors (without adequate recovery periods), estrogenic influences from foods, plastics, and pesticides, and deficiencies that trigger unfavorable cascades (such as sodium deficiency, causing your kidneys to activate the RAAS pathway as a compensation mechanism).[1]

When these environmental inputs are not properly balanced through support of protective hormones, which is almost always the cause due to the oppositional nature of the hormone relationships, the slow burn begins, a downward spiral of physical degeneration.

While there are many hormones involved in the human stress response, in the interest of pursuing *leveraged thinking,* we're going to focus on improving the following, since this will create the biggest positive impact in the shortest period of time:

1. Cortisol
2. Estrogen
3. Adrenaline and Noradrenaline

Evolutionary programming has created an extremely efficient stress response system in your body, known as the sympathetic nervous system. This can be a double-edged sword in our modern world.

In the presence of a stressor, the amygdala, which is considered to be the "fear center" of the brain, quickly signals to the hypothalamus to trigger a signaling cascade through the pituitary to the adrenal glands. This pathway is known as the HPA axis.

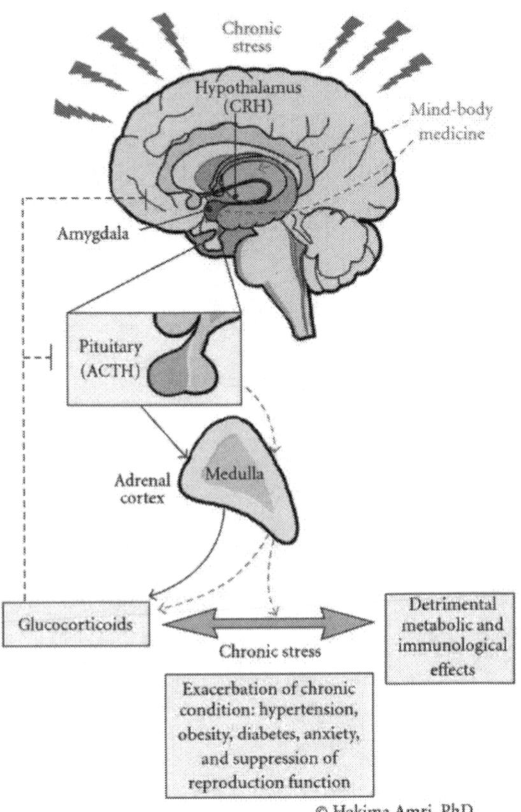

The pituitary gland, via the hormone ACTH (adrenocorticotropic hormone), tells the adrenal glands to push down the "gas pedal" by pumping cortisol and adrenaline into the bloodstream, which acutely heightens your senses, increases blood pressure, and triggers the release available glucose then stored fatty acids into the blood for extra energy.

Glucose, being readily available in acute stress situations, also happens to be in limited supply since it's needed for so many other important bodily functions. When cortisol is chronically elevated, glucose is quickly used up to fuel this "survival mechanism" and no longer available for important "thriving" processes like the brain's cognitive processes, reproductive processes, detoxification in the liver, and thyroid gland energy metabolism processes.

All resources are distributed to survival.

The problem is, chronic cortisol and adrenaline elevation inherently uses up preferred energy sources, and requires the body to switch to a survival metabolism, dumping stored fatty acids into the bloodstream, which creates unfavorable metabolic byproducts on the cellular level, such as lactic acid, and lowers overall CO2 production in the body which is needed for regenerative processes.

In modern chronic stress scenarios, we're not actually trying to "survive" in the primal sense of the word, but your body doesn't know the difference. It's wired to be extremely efficient at facilitating this stress response.

When your stress response is chronically engaged, with its resources being used to "survive," it creates a downward spiral of degeneration.

The good news: when you become aware of this, there are a lot of things you can do to stop it, by eliminating the Blockers that cause this chronic physiological stress, while introducing Activators that will support your protective hormones once again, to skew the hormonal balance back in your favor.

The Thermo Hormone Optimization Pyramid

In my first book, Master Your T, I outlined a diagram for readers on how to think about optimizing their testosterone production naturally, which I called the Masculine Optimization Pyramid. In designing the pyramid, it became obvious that people needed an easy way to visually understand how to do this, and since its advent, hundreds of thousands of men have used this diagram to rebalance their hormones naturally.

However, this pyramid framework is not just for men. It works for women as well, and it will help anyone rebalance their hormones naturally, namely decreasing stress hormones while increasing production of protective hormones.

I've redesigned the pyramid here for this purpose, and it's called the Thermo Hormone Optimization Pyramid.

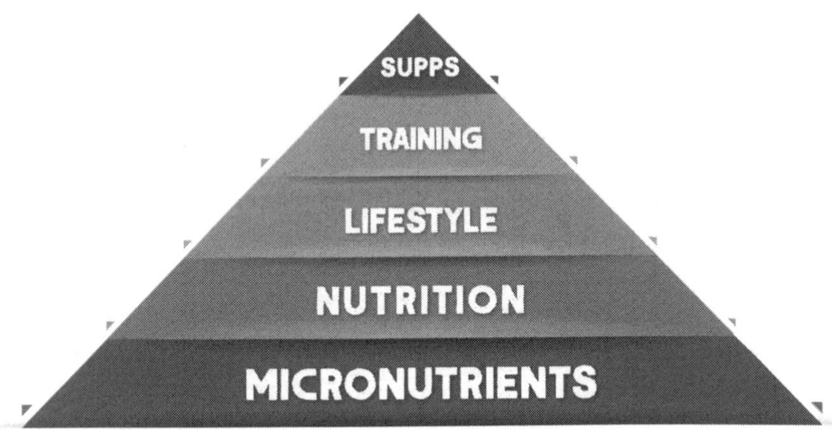

The order of importance goes from bottom to top, since you don't want to build your health on a shaky foundation.

Micronutrients are the key foundational element to rebalancing hormones. They are the raw materials your body needs to fuel every hormonal and metabolic process. When you're deficient in any vitamins, minerals, or amino acids, it throws hormones out-of-whack quickly. Therefore this needs to be the first thing you focus on.

Moving up the pyramid, nutrition becomes vitally important, mainly as a way to support your micronutrient levels, gut health (in order to absorb those micronutrients and facilitate proper neuronal signaling to the brain), and provide your body with the right macronutrients to thrive.

Nutrition is a very easy thing to manipulate. Simply eat foods that help your body function better, and stop eating things that hurt your body.

Next, we have Lifestyle implications. Inside this middle part of the pyramid you can include things like stress management techniques, sexual health practices, and eliminating exposure to estrogenic chemicals in your personal care products.

After Micronutrients, Nutrition, and Lifestyle are optimized, it's important to include proper exercise: physical activities that skew the hormonal balance in your favor, away from chronic cortisol activities (such as endurance training), toward anabolic activities (such as weight training) and restorative activities (such as walking or hiking).

The human body needs to be in motion. Researchers have demonstrated that without physical movement, the body starts to show signs of prediabetes in as little as 48 hours.[2]

And finally, the least important but still very useful top of the pyramid is strategic supplementation. Many people try to use supplements as a replacement, or shortcut, to substitute in place of the other levels of the pyramid. This typically doesn't serve them very well because the foundational levels of the pyramid are more profoundly impactful to your health. When your nutrition is poor, for example, supplementation can only help so much.

It's at the top because it is most useful to either aid the other levels of the pyramid, for example providing additional micronutrients to overcome deficiencies or using certain herbs for stress management lifestyle adjustments, or to use as a final "cherry on top" in terms of helping to truly optimize your performance once you address everything else underneath it.

If you optimize all of these levels of the Thermo Pyramid using the suggestions throughout this book you will rebalance your hormones and quickly restore the Thermo State of health back into your body.

CHAPTER EIGHT

CONTROL INFLAMMATION

THE LAW OF FIRE

Some inflammation can be good, with temperance, but most is bad. Without a clear understanding of what causes inflammation in your body, it will be difficult to control. Awareness is the first step toward Understanding. For most people, a systemic inflammatory response becomes chronic long before they take positive action to correct the issues causing it. The important thing to be aware of, is that it is indeed a "response," meaning there is a cause-effect relationship, and the inflammation can be moderated by identifying and eliminating the culprit stressor and introducing good "activators" into your body to quell the inflammatory response.

"Fire is the principle of all things. Conflict of opposites is a permanent state of all things."

Heraclitus

In *The Principia (1687)*, Isaac Newton's seminal work on the mathematical exploration of Nature, he states that *"To any action there is always an opposite and equal reaction; in other words, the actions of two bodies upon each other are always equal and always opposite in direction."*

I've found it helpful to remember, in the search for the truth about the body's operations, that nothing escapes the law of cause and effect; nothing is free. Nature is in a constant state of compensating, and the human body is not exempt from this reality.

Inflammation is the body's chief compensatory response to chemical stress.

The main macro process of opposing forces within your body is most easily understood as **regeneration** versus **degeneration**, and the oppositional nature between the two is almost entirely influenced by environmental factors: the inputs that either allow for the cells to coherently regenerate, or to dissonantly degenerate.

Inflammation, with the right element of control, is a natural part of regeneration, a process known as hormesis. Hormesis is the impetus for adaptation, and the subsequent development of growth and increased strength within the system. Hormetic stress is especially important in physical training, mitochondrial adaptations, and the maintenance of homeostasis (which is itself a demonstration of the body's innate drive to balance).

On the other hand, inflammation when uncontrolled, drives degeneration. Cellular dissonance caused by inflammatory reactions manifests in systemic dysfunction in tissues, organs, and organ systems.

As the body seeks homeostasis, the continual environmental input of inflammatory "blockers" compels it to find resources from within (since they're not being provided externally), in order to balance this degeneration, pulling micronutrients from important storage areas with inherently limited supplies.

Inflammation can ultimately be fatal.

Understand it if you want to improve your health.

The Chicken And The Egg

In 2012, the pioneering physiologist *Dr. Raymond Peat*, PhD from the University of Oregon, wrote about an illuminating observation regarding the nature of the effect of inflammation on aging (degeneration) in an organism by investigating the patterns seen in the brain development of different birds, relative to their gestational environment.[1]

The chicken egg, when incubated with heat from the mother hen, is a self-contained environment with all of the resources necessary for the development of a healthy baby chick, including glucose and nutrient-dense yolk. Brain growth stops when the chick embryo has consumed all of the available glucose within the egg, and needs to switch to consuming the fat of the yolk.

Chickens are known as *precocial* birds, meaning the chicks are completely developed when hatched, and therefore do not require further attention or care from the parent to survive into adulthood.

In September of 1979, researchers Zamenhof and Ahmad conducted a study on the influence of external injection of micronutrients into the developing brains of baby chickens while still inside the egg.[2]

Zamenhof and Ahmad injected several different types of amino acids into the brains of chick embryos and measured brain weight, DNA content, and protein content. They noted that several variations of the amino acid tryptophan severely inhibited brain development due to excess production of serotonin, while the introduction of glycine, which converts into glucose, stimulated significant brain growth.

They concluded that *"brain weight and DNA were found to be significantly correlated with blood glucose level"* and that *"early brain growth might be manipulated in both directions (inhibition or stimulation) by addition of proper nutrients during the sensitive period of neuronal proliferation."*

The positive influence of gestational glucose on brain development of the embryo has long been observed in many species, including humans. Results highlight the reality that glucose availability leads to larger brain sizes and increased neuron count in the newborn.

So in theory, while the mother chicken provides an adequate environment for the development of the embryo, it's not perfect, as evidenced when you compare the chicken to other species of birds, such as crows, parrots, and owls.

These altricial bird species are born in conditions more similar to humans. They require care from the mother in order to survive early stages of life, and have a steady access to additional sources of glucose, and therefore their brains, like human brains, continue to develop beyond birth.[3]

The differences in behavior between altricial birds and precocial birds is striking.

Parrots, for example, are considered to be highly intelligent and can live to be over 100 years old, and they can talk! Altricial birds are the only other animals that can produce human language. For example, the African Grey Parrot has such a highly developed speech ability, that it can mimic up to 1000 human words, and has been shown in captivity to be able to actually comprehend what it is saying much of the time, which gives it the ability to communicate with humans in a conversation.

Crows and ravens, also highly intelligent, can live between 10-60 years old (depending on environment), with the longest lifespan observed at 59 years for a captive pet crow named Tata from Bearsville, NY.[4]

Owls also generally have extended life spans up to 15 years, depending on species. One Great Horned Owl is known to have lived for 29 years.[5]

Altricial birds exhibit highly intelligent behavior patterns due to not only their more developed brains, but also because of their vulnerability and dependence upon parental care for early-stage survival, which acts an adaptive stress.

Artificial Intelligence researchers use the altricial-precocial spectrum as a model for the development of machine learning algorithms. Computer scientist Aaron Sloman and cognitive scientist Dr. Jackie Chappell from the University of Birmingham published a paper in 2005, establishing their theory that robot learning requires 2 key factors for altricial development, specifically:

1. Unpredictability: characterized in animals chiefly by the need to hunt unpredictable prey, as opposed to grazing or foraging

2. New Niches: characterized by the need for rapid adaptation and recalibration

... both of which highlight the need for rapid development of advanced intelligence for survival, dependent on the ability to learn and adapt to the environment quickly because of certain stimuli altricial species are commonly exposed to compared to precocial ones.

Birds have naturally high metabolic rates, evidenced by average body temperatures in the range of 110°F. Inside the egg, a precocial bird quickly burns through the available nutrient resources due to this high rate of energy consumption and needs. Its brain stops developing when glucose is no longer available.

Altricial birds generally have longer life spans and higher intelligence levels than precocial birds due to the combination of this high metabolic rate coupled with more glucose availability during early development, and the exposure to unpredictable environmental stimuli which require the development of rapid skill-learning for survival, a form of hormetic stress that makes the altricial animal more capable over time.

The development of not just these birds, but of all organisms, depends on the interplay between their environment and their bodies. The same is true of our cells.

Inflammation is environmental.

Over time, inflammation changes the way your body can operate, namely how effectively it can regenerate, or heal itself. This is due to internal shifts in resource availability, like nutrients, that the body needs for regenerative processes.

You'll notice that, in children and teenagers, the body can heal itself quite quickly after injury, due to a higher regenerative capacity. Over time, as the body is exposed to an increasing amount of inflammatory environmental "blockers," it has a decreasingly effective ability to recover.

The build up of inflammation inside your body is responsible for this, and you experience an increase in degeneration as you age, and eventually lose the regenerative ability entirely, resulting in death.

The inflammation response inside the body is characterized mainly by triggering the release of compounds known as inflammatory cytokines, which are catabolic, such as the interleukins IL-1β, TNFα, IL-6, IL-15, IL-17, and IL-18.

However, to highlight the opposing nature of regenerative and degenerative inflammation, it's important to understand that the body also has a host of anti-inflammatory interleukins such as IL-4, IL-10, and IL-13, which stimulate anabolic processes to restore order.[6]

When stimulation of inflammatory cytokines outpaces the anti-inflammatory cytokines, due to excessive environmental exposure to stressors, homeostasis is disrupted chronically, and destructive compensatory mechanisms kick in.

Other inflammatory cytokines that have been linked to cellular degeneration, discovered in much higher concentrations in adults compared to fetuses, are PDGF, TGF, IGF-1,[7] and bFGF, as well as prostaglandins.[8]

Prostaglandins are formed from the synthesis of the polyunsaturated fats linoleic acid and arachidonic acid.[9] Exposure to these supposedly "essential fatty acids" (see the *EAT SUGAR & DON'T EAT PUFA* chapters) is entirely diet-dependent, and therefore entirely within your control.

In the womb, the only possible way for the developing fetus to be exposed to these fatty acids is via the mother's dietary habits, and researchers have found that baby weights are negatively correlated with maternal exposure to these inflammatory polyunsaturated fatty acids.[10] The same researchers discovered that prenatal learning and memory are significantly retarded by exposure to PUFA in the womb.[11]

Monocytes, a type of white blood cell that are important for immune system adaptation, especially in the developing fetus, are killed off in the umbilical cord with exposure to polyunsaturated fats,[12] which greatly compromises the child's ability to control inflammation properly as it continues to develop. Yet, curiously, the US Food and Drug Administration has approved the use of manufactured additive forms of these harmful fatty acids into baby formulas.[13]

Degenerative inflammation has become commonplace, a *way of life* for most people, mostly due to our modern environment, dietary habits & subsequent chronic nutrient deficiencies, and unregulated stressors.

This creates a steady decline in the body's ability to heal itself.

Naturally, you start to experience symptoms of this degeneration over time, which most people chock up to "getting old."

Inflammation is blamed for causing everything from obesity, to heart disease, high blood pressure, arthritis, asthma, ulcers, oral diseases, celiac, gut issues such as IBS, Crohn's, and ulcerative colitis, autoimmune diseases in general, and so much more.

However, does just pointing to "inflammation" as the cause really help anyone with these issues? No, it doesn't. Inflammation is the first stage symptom, merely a response from your body warning you of a deeper true cause - it's the *effect* in the ubiquitous cause-effect matrix happening all around us, all the time.

I'm far more interested in unearthing true causes of the myriad negative biological effects we experience in the inflammatory milieu.

When you understand the true causes, you can actually do something to help yourself eliminate the "blockers" that strip your regenerative abilities. This is where rubber meets the road.

How To Control Inflammation

The chief molecular indicators of degenerative inflammation are inflammatory cytokines and prostaglandins.

You can control both of them pretty easily. This is not a black box, as many people would like you to believe.

I recommend controlling degenerative inflammation by altering your dietary habits, and I've also found that, in acute inflammation scenarios, using certain exogenous compounds, namely specific supplement extracts and amino acids can be extremely helpful and fast-acting to lower systemic inflammation.

If we start with the most basic requirement for controlling inflammation in your body, it all comes down to heat production: your metabolism.

As I've discussed in a lot of detail in this book, and will discuss more, your metabolic rate (easily measured via waking body temperature) is the indicator that, not only is a high amount of energy flowing easily through your cells, but that your hormones are balanced, and unfavorable anti-metabolic byproducts are limited and don't have much influence in creating any sort of cellular dissonance.

You want your cells to consume as much oxygen, and produce as much CO_2 as possible.

CO_2, as a metabolic byproduct, signals to neighboring cells in concert, fueling cellular coherence as a positive feedback loop upward through the structured systems of the body, which creates more order in those systems, and more energy flow through them.

CO_2 is used in medical settings, such as intensive care units and in surgeries,[14] as a reliable way to shut down inflammatory cytokines and prostaglandin synthesis,[15-16] and can reverse symptoms of "leaky gut," by aiding in restoring the structural integrity of the intestinal wall.[17]

A high ratio of CO_2 to oxygen has been widely observed to have a stem cell-like regenerative effect in living tissue.

Not only have researchers discovered very high CO_2 to oxygen ratios in animals such as salamanders and other amphibians like the Xenopus,[18] which possess the ability to regenerate brain tissue, retina, spinal cord, and even entire limbs,[19] but they've also measured high CO_2 to oxygen ratios in specific human tissues and organs that have regenerative abilities, such as inside of the mouth, bones, bone marrow, thymus gland, thyroid gland, liver *(in the presence of adequate thyroid hormone)*, and adrenal cortex, all of which can regenerate tissue without scarring or fibrosis.

One amazing example of the human body's ability to regenerate tissue and bone, is the regeneration of fingertips after amputation. Studying this phenomenon gives us a lot of insight into the power of CO_2 production in living tissue.

Conventional wisdom in the medical community holds the belief that the ability for the body to regenerate fingertips rapidly declines with age after childhood,[20] however is "age" really the issue, or are there other factors in play, like cytokines?

In fact, a study conducted on (mean age) 50 year old adults demonstrated significant ability to regenerate fingertips if certain conditions were present: namely, CO_2 and nerve growth factor BDNF.[21]

They found that the ability to regenerate the tissue was dependent on enclosing the fingertip in an occlusive environment, which allows for humidity to increase the CO_2 levels present around the injured tissue in a local microenvironment, and subsequently triggers release of growth factors like BDNF, HGF, and EGF.

In fingertip regeneration studies, inflammatory cytokines are highly expressive in the first week, due to the traumatic injury, then in the right conditions, anti-inflammatory cytokines are more highly expressed during the second week after injury, indicating a positive shift in the body's healing response, which leads to oftentimes a full eventual regeneration of not just the bone, marrow, and skin, but also an entire well-formed fingernail.[22]

Another key element in the progression of inflammatory degeneration, commonly expressed in autoimmune diseases, is the decreasing ability for the body to clear apoptotic, or dead, cells. Apoptosis is programmed cell death, and is a normal process in living tissue, required for proper growth and development.

Cellular clearance that takes place inside our bodies is required in order to reinforce healthy systems and prune unhealthy ones, akin to a gardener pruning the dead branches from plants in order to keep the overall plant healthy.

Apoptosis, and clearance of apoptotic cells, is an energy-dependent process.[23] Energetic dysfunction leads to a decline in clearance.

Active thyroid hormone, T3, is necessary for the proper functioning of this clearance process[24] of dead cells out of the degenerating tissue, which allows for the formation of new tissue.

But with excess inflammatory cytokine and prostaglandin activity in the tissue, indicating degenerative inflammation, the body loses its ability to clear these dead cells. For example, a study published in the Journal of Clinical and Experimental

Immunology demonstrated that radiation-induced inflammation causes a significant loss in the animals' ability to clear dead cells, which leads to rapid onset of autoimmune disease symptoms.[25]

This is seen in the liver as well,[26] with the liberation of free fatty acids causing significant degeneration in liver tissue. The researchers in that particular study concluded that the single most important factor in aging-related degeneration is the disruption of the glucose metabolism and the resulting hormone imbalance. They also noted that dietary calorie restriction could slow the decline.

This, once again, brings us back to the nature of polyunsaturated fatty acids as a consistently disruptive force driving degeneration in the body.

Foods And Supplements That Help You Control Inflammation Naturally

1. *Glycine:*

The perfect place to start on our hunt for natural compounds that can help us lower degenerative inflammation, is to examine inflammatory cytokines, namely what compounds are involved in their reaction process.

Ultimately, the restoration of real health - *Thermo* - back into your body will almost always end with micronutrients, such as amino acids.

It turns out that the inflammatory cytokine reaction increases in prevalence with glycine deficiencies.[27] This makes a lot of sense because glycine has an inhibitory action,[28] and via glycine-gated chloride channels[29] in immune cells,[30] can temper many inflammatory cytokines, including IL-6.[31]

The important thing to understand about amino acids is the fact that in our modern culturally-normal diets, especially in the Western world, we tend to eat a lot of muscle meat, and eschew meats such as organs, as well as collagen-rich connective tissue and bones from the animal.

This leads to an amino acid imbalance over time in your body, causing deficiencies in amino acids that your body needs for important cellular processes while increasing circulating amounts of other amino acids into a surplus, which can ultimately be harmful.

For example, muscle meats, which do contain small amounts of glycine, are much higher in methionine, an amino acid that gets converted into the universal methyl donor SAMe. Your body has innate methionine-regulating mechanisms to get rid of excess methionine, however these mechanisms are dependent on the presence of adequate glycine to operate properly.[32]

Without enough glycine, and especially with high amounts of circulating methionine, your body has a difficult time creating glutathione, the "master antioxidant" that is so crucial for regulating inflammation and your immune system in general.

The liver cannot keep up with the demand of trying to synthesize endogenous glycine via the glycine-serine pathway because you eventually run out of the "raw materials" involved in the process. Excess methionine sends your system into overdrive, trying to constantly get rid of it.

This results in widespread degenerative inflammation in your body. Quite simply, consuming more glycine can stop this.

And luckily, glycine is quite easy to get in high amounts, and very affordable. I personally consume between 10-15g of glycine per day from UMZU collagen and grass-fed bone broth, adding the collagen protein to fruit smoothies, which is important because I also regularly eat a pound of grass-fed beef or game muscle meat (elk, buffalo, venison) daily, which contains more methionine than glycine. You need to balance the amino acid ratio.

All of this biology may sound quite complicated, but when a basic understanding of the need for these important nutrients is in place, taking action on it is surprisingly easy. I recommend building regular glycine consumption into your daily habits.

Glycine is widely studied. It's been shown to help improve diabetic symptoms,[33] heal wounds and stop tumor growth,[34] protect the body from alcohol-related and dietary inflammation,[35] increase lifespan and help regulate cholesterol properly,[36] protect against neurological and organ damage,[37] lower endotoxin levels,[38] stop acid reflux,[39] and reverse fatty liver issues and liver damage.[40]

It's incredibly useful to your body, to say the least. Eat more glycine.

2. *Turmeric root:*

You've likely heard of turmeric. The NIH has a large body of documented human research on the benefits of using turmeric for a variety of reasons.[41] Turmeric is a widely used root powder around the world, and has been in use for thousands of years, especially in its native regions such as India, Asia, and Central America.

Turmeric is used as both a spice and a natural anti-inflammatory supplement ingredient, due to its distinct flavor and curcuminoid content, respectively.

One of the most common uses for turmeric is in pain management. In fact, put head-to-head with Ibuprofen in studies, turmeric was shown to be more effective at reducing pain.[42]

Another study showed that rheumatoid arthritis patients who took a natural turmeric supplement saw greater improvements than patients given Voltaren, diclofenac sodium.

In a 2016 study,[43] researchers concluded that curcumin may be effective for treating joint-related pain. The Arthritis Foundation also supports the use of turmeric for relieving arthritic pain.[44]

Blood clotting is a common symptom of degenerative inflammation. Turmeric has anti-thrombotic properties. Curcumin may reduce stroke and heart attack by preventing clogged arteries. It does this by inhibiting platelet aggregation, or the clumping of blood platelets that lead to clotting. Turmeric's effect as an anticoagulant was confirmed in a 2012 study.[45]

Curcumin is known to interact with neurotrophic factors (NTF) in the brain. NTFs are a form of peptides that aid in the growth and maturity of brain neurons. Studies show that curcumin induces NTF production and may help treat various central nervous system disorders.[46]

Studies also suggest that turmeric may be more effective for treating depression than fluoxetine, the generic form of Prozac.

In one study,[47] 60 human subjects diagnosed with depression were given curcumin, fluoxetine, or a combination of the two. After six weeks, the curcumin group reported just as much improvement in mood as the fluoxetine group. A more extensive study with 108 male subjects yielded similar results.[48]

Turmeric contains natural COX-2 inhibitors. COX-2 is an

enzyme that aids in the production of the fatty acid prostanoid. This compound is a primary mediator of inflammation.

One study also found both turmeric and ginger to be effective for inhibiting cytokine production.[49]

Curcumin is especially known to treat the skin condition scabies, where microscopic mites called Sarcoptes Scabiei burrow under your skin. The eggs and waste they leave behind causes itchiness, rashes, and bumps.

In one study, 814 subjects with scabies used a topical turmeric treatment. 97% experienced relief within three to 15 days.[50]

Turmeric, in fact, is an old folk remedy in Indian Ayurvedic medicine for killing skin mites. Scabies is especially common in confined areas where skin-to-skin contact is commonplace, like in India due to the dense population in urban areas.

3. *Boswellia Serrata:*

Boswellia is more commonly known as frankincense, with a rich ancient history. It happens to be incredibly useful for tempering inflammation, especially with respect to arthritic pain symptoms.

An extensive 2011 report concluded that frankincense may be beneficial as an anti-inflammatory agent.[51] This was supported by a 2015 study that showed strong evidence for frankincense as an inflammation suppressor.[52] That's not all; a systematic review analyzing 47 studies on frankincense showed that the compound was effective for treating both rheumatoid and osteoarthritis.[53] On top of that, the research also concluded that frankincense was effective for treating other conditions, such as colitis and Crohn's disease.

How does frankincense bring down inflammation? It actually does this through multiple pathways. One way is by inhibiting the production of pro-inflammatory cytokines. Cytokines refer to a number of small proteins that play an active role in cell signaling. They're secreted by the immune system and interact with other cells. Depending on the type of cytokine, that interaction may be good or bad for the body. Just as there are pro-inflammatory cytokines that create disease and illness, there are also anti-inflammatory cytokines that help the body.

One study showed that frankincense suppresses pro-inflammatory cytokine production in joint cartilage.[54]

Furthermore, frankincense also contains a compound known as acetyl-11-keto boswellic acid (AKBA). Studies show that this substance inhibits an inflammatory enzyme known as 5-lipoxygenase.[55]

On top of that, frankincense is also known for boosting the immune system. This is especially good news for sufferers of rheumatoid arthritis. Remember that rheumatoid is an autoimmune disease caused by an abnormal immune response.

Frankincense corrects this response by promoting white blood cell production and improving your body's natural response to inflammation and foreign pathogens.

Store shelves are lined with nonsteroidal anti-inflammatory drugs (NSAID) like Ibuprofen, Motrin, and Advil for relieving arthritis pain. As with any other synthetic medication, there are side effects. Users of such products have reported nausea, stomach cramps, diarrhea, increased perspiration, and swelling.

There is also the risk of overdosing on NSAIDs and causing serious health problems. Regular use of Ibuprofen has actually been linked to stomach ulcers and gastrointestinal bleeding. The likelihood of this occurring depends on frequency of use and your sensitivity. If you become reliant on the drugs and take it every day just to manage the pain, then you up the odds of the NSAIDs causing serious damage. Stomach ulcers are no laughing matter. According to data, roughly one in 13 cases result in death.[56] The mortality rate increases to one in five when NSAIDs enter the equation.

4. *Bromelain:*

Bromelain is a protein-digesting *(proteolytic)* enzyme that is known for its ability to ease digestion by reducing inflammation. It's found mainly in pineapple, particularly in the flesh and stem.

On a molecular level, bromelain is made up of several compounds, such as cellulase, peroxidase, glucosidase and protease inhibitors. Though the medicinal properties of bromelain are just starting to receive modern scientific validity, it has long been used medicinally in Hawaii and parts of South America.

The studies behind bromelain as a digestive enhancer are strong. One research study suggests that the enzyme may inhibit the production of inflammatory cytokines.[57]

Another study arrived at similar conclusions. The researchers suggest that plant-based proteolytic enzymes like bromelain may be a powerful aid for alleviating various digestive disorders.[58]

Athletes and post-surgery patients are also increasingly turning to bromelain as a natural alternative. A study in 2004 revealed that bromelain is effective for treating pain from an ankle injury. In the trial, 73.7 percent of subjects that supplemented with bromelain for seven days reported less pain.[59]

Another study showed that bromelain reduced pain and swelling in patients recovering from post-operative surgery to heal a fracture injury.[60] One study on asthmatic mice showed that bromelain may reduce allergic reactions that cause the airways to swell and become inflamed.[61]

The immune support may also alleviate associating symptoms, such as nasal decongestion and itchy eyes. It's believed that bromelain suppresses certain dendritic cells known to trigger asthma.

In one study, patients recovering from nasal surgery saw a vast improvement in symptoms after taking all-natural bromelain tablets. Subjects also reported zero side effects. Like many other ailments, sinus congestion occurs as a result of the nasal passageways flaring up from inflammation. Bromelain's inflammation-reducing properties clear up the passageways.

One study concluded that bromelain shows promise for treating arthritis pain in the knees and shoulders. The study also concluded that it reduced acute pain by up to 60 percent in patients suffering from pain in the spinal region.[62]

5. *Olive leaf extract:*

Olive polyphenols and oleuropein are the components in olive leaf extract that offer numerous health benefits. Studies show that olive leaf extract possesses anti-inflammatory properties and protects against DNA damage that is caused by free radicals among numerous other benefits that are thought to contribute to longer lifespans among those who consume olive leaf extract.[63]

Research has shown that olive leaf extract can improve the lipid profile and help with glycemic control in those who have been diagnosed with diabetes.[64]

A study conducted showed that olive leaf extract can help regulate blood pressure as well as cholesterol levels.[65] Further research shows that the number of thromboembolic diseases are on the rise. Thromboembolisms are incidences in which a piece of a blood clot breaks off and travels through the bloodstream and blocks a different vessel. The study shows that olive leaf extract has anti-thrombotic effects.[66]

The polyphenols in olive leaf extract have been shown to have anti-inflammatory effects in individuals who have experienced trauma of the bone marrow.[67] A separate study also concluded that olive leaf extract has anti-inflammatory in various metabolic pathways in the human body.[68]

Olive leaf extract is also beneficial to the skin. Studies show that when applied to wounds, it speeds up the healing process.[69] The same study showed that it also has anti-aging effects when used as a cream on the skin, due to the regenerative stimulation it provides to the tissue.

6. *Cannabidiol:*

There is a rapidly expanding amount of research on cannabinoids like cannabidiol (CBD), all indicating pretty impressive benefits of CBD for inflammation, typically looking at inflammation biomarkers (indicators) and positive improvements when subjects use CBD or Hemp Extract over the control groups. Using CBD oil for inflammation is becoming increasingly more common as awareness around cannabis increases.

The body of research will no doubt continue to grow as more funding pours into this space, and as public interest continues to rise. Also, when cannabis becomes federally legal in the United States, then we will really see a large influx of research funding into the therapeutic uses of the plant.

One of the most promising areas of study for natural inflammation-reduction has involved the endocannabinoid system, namely CB1 and CB2 receptor activation which are G-protein-coupled receptor sites and the ligands that activate them.

Cannabidiol has a distinct way of interacting with the endocannabinoid system that appears very promising for therapeutic applications with relation to inflammation.[69] Much of the research in this area regarding inflammation is correlated with arthritis,[70] Type 1 and 2 diabetes,[71] atherosclerosis, Alzheimer's,[72] hypertension,[73] metabolic syndrome,[74] depression,[75] and neuropathy.[76]

Neuropathy is caused by microglia (the most common form of cellular immune defense) activation in the brain and spinal cord, which triggers the release of the cytokines interleukin-6 (IL-6), interleukin-1β (IL-1β), and tumor necrosis factor-α (TNFα), which put into simple terms, ***are pro-inflammatory molecules.***

The causes of neuropathic pain itself are poorly understood outside of this basic biological reaction. However, neuropathy pain is present in nearly all common forms of disease such as diabetes, cancer, autoimmune diseases, and MS.[77]

In a mouse model, CBD was demonstrated to alleviate heat sensitivity and allodynia (neuropathy pain) significantly.[77]

Two other studies demonstrated a very impressive calming of the immune system microglia/cytokine response along with promising anti-inflammatory improvements in patients with rheumatoid arthritis.[78-79]

By reducing insulin resistance and increasing insulin sensitivity, CBD was found in two separate research studies to reduce the initiation of diabetes and the development of latent diabetes in diabetes prone subjects.[71, 80] The super cool thing about this, is that this result was also accompanied by a shift from a pro-inflammatory cytokine response to an anti-inflammatory response.

Major effectors of β-cell death in type 1 diabetes are various free radicals and oxidant species, including NO, and infiltrating macrophages are one source of high concentrations of NO and inflammatory cytokines that further enhance NO and ROS formation.[81]

CBD oil has been shown in multiple studies to block ROS-induced up-regulation of surface adhesion molecules due to high blood glucose levels, which has preserved the barrier function of the endothelial cells,[82] thus restricting those pesky free radicals and other oxidant species from infiltrating the β-cells.[83]

A large body of evidence in recent years has implicated this similar cytokine inflammatory response[84] with depression in humans.[85] The most convincing explanation is that the presence of excessive free radicals and oxidant species like free fatty acids triggers the microglial cells to signal the release of the pro-inflammatory cytokines, which leads to depressive symptoms.

CBD has been reported to aid in calming this response in medical research.

This study specifically assessed the antidepressant and mood-elevating activity of CBD oil finding that its effect appeared to be dose dependent.[86]

This study posits that this antidepressant effect of CBD oil is likely due to activation of 5-HT1A receptors in the brain.[87]

Research in this area of CBD and inflammation is quickly evolving, and many of these papers I've cited here have put forward some very interesting theories surrounding promising therapies for people with diseases characterized by inflammation response due to microglial cell activation and the resulting pro-inflammatory cytokine increase.

7. *Niacinamide:*

Vitamin B3 as niacinamide is an important vitamin that is used in many ways by your body. Niacinamide plays an important role in protecting your thyroid gland against excess oxidative stress, including inhibiting the release of free fatty acids, which is one of the key causes of thyroid dysfunction.[88] Vitamin B3 boosts energy production in the cells and helps support metabolic rate via proper thyroid functioning.

Niacinamide helps balance the thyroid and overcome or prevent either hypothyroidism or hyperthyroidism. It's important to have all of the right vitamins, minerals and amino acids in the right forms and dosages in your body for a healthy thyroid, since they all interact with one another and help balance each other out.

Focus on these Thermo foods to get your daily requirements of niacinamide:

- **Chicken** — 1 cup: 19.2 milligrams (96 percent DV)
- **Liver** — 1 slice: 11.9 milligrams (60 percent DV)
- **Sardines** — 1 can: 4.8 milligrams (24 percent DV)
- **Grass-Fed Beef** — 3 ounces: 4.4 milligrams (22 percent DV)
- **Mushrooms** — 1 cup: 2.5 milligrams (13 percent DV)
- **Avocado** — 1 cup, cubed: 2.6 milligrams (13 percent DV)
- **Sweet Potatoes** — 1 medium: 1.7 milligrams (8 percent DV)

And if you want niacinamide from supplement form, I recommend pairing it with L-tyrosine, copper, selenium, and a good iodine supplement from kelp extract as well, since they work together synergistically in helping overcome thyroid imbalance.

8. *Vitamin B6:*

Not only is B6 crucial in the synthesis of GABA,[89] your body's chief inhibitory neurotransmitter, but it also has been shown to lower systemic homocysteine levels.[90] Homocysteine is synthesized from methionine, and in high amounts will radically increase degenerative inflammation.

Excess homocysteine levels are correlated with heart attacks, blood clotting,[91] early pregnancy loss,[92] neural tube defects,[93] and strokes.

Elevation of homocysteine is highly linked to serious neuropsychiatric issues, such as schizophrenia,[94] bipolar disorder, depression, anxiety, and Alzheimer's.[95-96] Dr. William Walsh highlights the importance of correcting B6 deficiencies in his book *Nutrient Power.*[97] Through analysis of 100,000s of patients over his career, in both clinical and laboratory settings, Dr. Walsh has identified predictable biochemical patterns present in all of the aforementioned neuropsychiatric conditions, the most common of which is vitamin B6 deficiencies.

CHAPTER NINE

LOWER SEROTONIN

THE LAW OF CHEMICAL WARFARE

A healthy body requires balanced neurotransmitter production. Modern marketing for antidepressant drugs has been so effective at co-opting not just the medical community, but also the alternative health circles (calling it the "happy hormone" even though it's not a hormone at all), regulating bodies, and the popular media, that most people now believe that they're serotonin deficient. This could not be further from the truth, in fact most evidence points to population-wide excess of serotonin, and this serotonin overload is responsible for myriad devastating physical and psychological dysfunctions. The easy shorthand narrative about serotonin deficiency causing depression is not just lazy, it is fraudulent: completely inaccurate. Excess serotonin leads to overproduction of stress hormones such as estrogen, cortisol, and prolactin and conditions the human body & mind to "learned helplessness," a phenomenon that has been demonstrated in animal research to trigger disturbingly acute suicidal behaviors. You don't need more serotonin, you need less! You must work to lower serotonin production while increasing natural production of vital neurotransmitters such as dopamine, acetylcholine, and GABA to restore balance to your gut and brain, which will give you the feelings of well-being, energy, and clarity you're searching for.

"Prozac is incredibly easy to prescribe. You can teach a chimpanzee to prescribe it."

-*Psychopharmacologist*, **New York Magazine** article in 1989

Only ten years after Prozac, the blockbuster "antidepressant" drug, was approved for sale in the US by the FDA, the Boston Globe reported that an estimated 50,000 people had committed suicide because of using the drug.

Prozac acts in the brain as a selective serotonin reuptake inhibitor, meaning it blocks the reabsorption of serotonin that is sent out from the presynaptic neuron, leaving more serotonin to flood the space between the two communicating neurons, also known as the synaptic cleft. This mechanism of action allows for more serotonin to bind to the postsynaptic neuron's receptor sites, propagating the action of serotonin further than it would normally go in a healthy brain.

The term *antidepressant* that drug companies are now using to market this class of SSRI pharmaceuticals, is a misnomer: it's highly misleading. As I will explain in more depth, increasing the action and amount of circulating serotonin has the exact opposite of an antidepressant effect, which explains the rapid uptick in suicides following the introduction of SSRIs into the market in the 1990s.

In fact, the BGA, Germany's food and drug administration, refused to approve Prozac in 1987, just a few years before Prozac's manufacturer Lilly brought it to the US; German regulators were disturbed by the results of human trials where subjects who were previously non-suicidal experienced a 5-fold increase in suicide rates and suicide attempts, compared to when treated with older MAOI antidepressant drugs (which had expired patents at the time).

But let's wind the clocks back for a minute, because there is a lot more to this story than most people know...

How did we get to this point? Why does everyone believe serotonin is the "happy hormone" that we all need more of, even in the face of so much damning evidence to the contrary? And why are serotonin agonists still being so widely prescribed by physicians?

The answer lies hidden deep in the history of lysergic acid diethylamide, yes... LSD.

LSD: The Antiserotonin Agent

On April 16th 1943, swiss scientist Albert Hofmann was resynthesizing a stimulant chemical that he'd discovered years prior by adding a functional group to a compound he extracted from a fungus in 1938, but had temporarily abandoned.

Accidentally absorbing some of the chemical through his fingertips, he had to lay down, and quickly experienced what he described as an extremely stimulated imagination.

"In a dreamlike state, with eyes closed, I perceived an uninterrupted stream of fantastic pictures, extraordinary shapes with intense, kaleidoscopic play of colors. After some two hours this condition faded away." - ***LSD: Mein Sorgenkind by Albert Hofmann***

Hofmann, who was ranked in 2007 as the #1 living genius of our time by the UK's *The Daily Telegraph,* had discovered LSD, and 3 days later, took the first full-dose acid trip.

The world was about to change.

Sandoz Laboratories, Hofmann's employer, introduced LSD as a drug treatment for schizophrenia and alcoholism in 1947 in Europe.

Soon thereafter, in the 1950s, things started getting weird.

According to public disclosure by president Gerald Ford in 1975 through the *Rockefeller Commission,* a federal investigation into illegal CIA activities, the CIA had purchased the entire world's supply of LSD from Sandoz Laboratories, and secretly introduced it into the US.

Their focus was on *mind control* experimentation, with the chief aim of finding drugs that could be used in clandestine operations in order to wipe a subject's mind clean so it could be reprogrammed.

For nearly a decade the CIA experimented on mental patients, prisoners, sex workers, CIA employees, military personnel, and even members of the general public, almost always without the subjects' consent or prior knowledge.

According to now declassified CIA documents,[1] the agency abandoned LSD experimentation in 1962 because it proved "too unpredictable" for achieving their mind control objective.

Less than a year later, Sandoz Laboratories' patents on LSD expired.

By this point, writers such as Aldous Huxley, Alan Watts, and Timothy Leary had begun openly advocating for the therapeutic usage of LSD and psilocybin, both potent antiserotonin compounds, for the exact opposite purpose of the CIA's programs – *to expand an individual's mental perception.*

After Leary and his research partner Richard Alpert, also known as Ram Dass, were very publicly fired from Harvard University in 1963 for their experiments on LSD and psilocybin, the '60s counterculture movement in the US started to pick up steam, with widespread use of psychedelic compounds in the general population, until 1968 when possession of LSD was made illegal by the federal government, then subsequently listed as a schedule 1 controlled narcotic by the United Nations in 1971.

Nixon's presidency from 1969 to 1974 marked an interesting time in the "War on Drugs," with the official establishment of the Drug Enforcement Agency (DEA), and a public declaration that "drug abuse" was *public enemy number one* in 1971.

Nixon is also quoted as saying that Timothy Leary is, "the most dangerous man in America."[2]

Leary, the inspiration for John Lennon's song "Come Together," was thrown in jail 36 times throughout his life, most often for marijuana possession and ultimately for escaping prison before being recaptured by federal agents. He eventually ended up in California's maximum security Folsom Prison in the cell adjacent to Charles Manson.

The two men reportedly had a conversation about LSD where Charles Manson is quoted as telling Leary, *"they took you off the streets, so I could continue the work,"* where Manson expressed frustration and difficulty understanding why Leary had never used LSD for mind control purposes, rather he advocated for it to help people expand their minds, quite the opposite.[3]

Manson, on the other hand, was well-known for performing methods similar to the CIA's original experiments on his

"Family" to psychologically program them before the infamous murder of Sharon Tate.

With such a huge focus on chemical-induced mind control by government agencies throughout this time, it may seem serendipitous that the 1950s and '60s also ushered in the first two generations of antidepressant pharmaceuticals, which could more accurately described as tranquilizers. Physicians began prescribing these drugs to patients across the US en masse.

It's important to understand this: ***LSD is a powerful serotonin antagonist.***

With disturbingly analogous similarities to the "Reefer Madness" tactics employed by the Federal Bureau of Narcotics in the 1930s, resulting in the federal ban of marijuana in 1937, the anti-LSD propaganda leading up to its prohibition in 1968 focused on claims that it induced homicidal violence.

> "LSD is a psychedelic drug which occasionally causes psychotic behavior in people who have NOT taken it."
>
> **- Timothy Leary**

The first 2 generations of antidepressant drugs weren't the only thing that rose in popularity during this time, but also specific serotonin-precursor supplements, namely the amino acid L-tryptophan, 5-HTP (5-hydroxytryptophan), and the hormone melatonin*.

**Dr. Richard Wurtmann, the MIT and Harvard doctor who discovered melatonin's hormone action in 1994, is quoted as saying that nobody should use melatonin as a dietary supplement due to known health risks associated with it. Yet, it continues to be sold over the counter, widely used by millions of men, women, and children.*

"Misconceptions about serotonin and melatonin and tryptophan, which are metabolically interrelated, have persisted, and it seems that the drug industry has exploited these mistakes to promote the "new generation" of psychoactive drugs as activators of serotonin responses. If LSD makes people go berserk, as the government claimed, then a product to amplify the effects of serotonin should make people sane." - ***Dr. Raymond Peat, PhD***

Serotonin itself wasn't officially discovered until 1935, when an Italian researcher named Vittorio Erspamer isolated a monoamine compound from enterochromaffin cells, which caused the intestinal walls to contract. He named this compound, "enteramine."

13 years later, researchers at the Cleveland Clinic discovered an amine in blood serum that appeared to act as a vasoconstricting agent. They named it "serotonin" (serum + tone).

In 1952, scientists finally realized that enteramine and serotonin were the same chemical.

That same year, MAOIs (monoamine oxidase inhibitors) were introduced by drug companies into the marketplace, alongside the "monoamine theory of depression," in an attempt to artificially raise circulating levels of monoamines like serotonin in the body.

90% of serotonin is produced in the gut, contrary to popular assumption that it is all in the brain. Your gut is called your "second brain," the enteric nervous system, for a reason: it contains roughly 500 million neurons.

Your gut-based enteric nervous system communicates neuronally to your brain via the spinal cord, and bacterially via production of certain gases to catalyze reactions and cascades within the body.

Messing with gut function, especially neuronally, is risky business.

Curiously timed alongside the "War On Drugs," the development of these serotonin-amplifying pharmaceuticals built unstoppable momentum in the public relations sector, and they were embraced by government regulators as the antidote to mind-opening drugs like LSD and psilocybin, the antiserotonin agents, which had already proven too unwieldy for them to control.

In 1950, two years before MAOIs were introduced to the general public, sociology researchers out of UC Berkeley published a seminal book entitled, *The Authoritarian Personality,* the contents of which set forth their theory that, based on a

Freudian developmental model, people developed either an "authoritarian" personality or "anti-authoritarian" personality, both of which have a biological basis.

Authoritarian personalities are characterized by harm avoidance behaviors, unquestioning submission to authority figures, passive-aggression, and extreme obedience, all behaviors shown in scientific research to correlate with high levels of serotonin.

Quite possibly the most extreme, and disturbing, examples of serotonin's ability to induce authoritarian personality behaviors can be seen in studies demonstrating "learned helplessness" in animals.

When exposed to excess serotonin levels, researchers can quite literally create *learned helplessness* in animals, which creates the perception of inescapable stress, pure hopelessness. Common studies demonstrate this with swimming scenarios, where the serotonin-animal is placed in a water maze and forced to swim. The non-serotonin exposed control animals will continue swimming, potentially even for hours in order to survive.

But when the serotonin-group animals are placed in the water maze, they exhibit signs of extreme stress within minutes and subsequently give up trying, allowing themselves to drown. They have no capacity whatsoever to cope with the stress.

Researchers think this type of learned helplessness occurs for several reasons:

1. High serotonin levels tend to trigger the production of a lot of lactic acid via glycolysis, which interferes directly with mitochondrial respiration, as I've discussed earlier in this book already. This slows the metabolic rate significantly, leaving the animal with diminished energy.
2. Panic reactions, extreme muscle pain, hypertension, and heart failure are all correlated with high serotonin levels.[4]

Anti-authoritarian personalities, on the other hand, are expressed through high dopamine levels and low serotonin, and are characterized in the individual through risk-taking behaviors, lack of obedience, and a disregard for authority figures.

It's logical why, on a population level, intelligence agencies, drug companies, and governments would be interested in declaring a war on antiserotonin drugs. The 1960s were famously known as the *"Counterculture Movement"* after all, and Timothy Leary was the figurehead, "the most dangerous man in America."

One interesting thing to note, is that after MAOIs were introduced in the 1950s, incidences of migraines spiked, especially in women. We now know why.[5] Estrogen is an endogenous MAOI itself. The estrogen stimulates an increased rate of serotonin production. The excess serotonin has a vasoconstrictive action, decreasing blood flow to the brain, while veins and capillaries on the surface of the brain swell with blood, causing intense migraines and cluster headaches.

MAOIs were eventually phased out of widespread use, mostly due to some pretty gnarly side effects in patients, but also likely due to patent expirations. Once a patent on a drug expires, it can no longer be controlled as a high priced "brand name" and generally becomes a generic, lower priced version of the same product.

With the serotonin-driven consumer beliefs deeply entrenched in our cultural psyche, drug companies developed a class of new drugs, with new patents, to work on amplifying serotonin: SSRIs.

SSRI drugs, such as Prozac, were released in the '90s alongside aggressive marketing about how your "depression is a deficiency in the happy hormone" and a lot of marketing around the idea of a "chemical imbalance" in your brain.

Branded as antidepressants, SSRIs commonly demonstrate the exact opposite effect in patients, triggering unnatural suicides at alarming rates, including in depressed patients who were not previously suicidal. This is indicative of learned helplessness.

SSRIs have been shown in ever-increasing mountains of research to cause serious side effects that mostly serve to make the patient's condition worse, including:

- Worsening of bipolar disorder due to negative neuroplastic changes[6]
- No improvements in major depression,[7] no difference between SSRIs and control after a year of treatment[8-12]

- Placebo provided better results in reducing suicide risk than SSRI[13]
- 50% failure in trials, but published by the FDA and touted as 94% effective[14]
- Increased incidence of anxiety disorders[15-16]
- Thyroid problems[17]
- Increased stress levels[18]
- Increased aggressive behavior[19]
- Alzheimer's risk[20]
- Mitochondrial dysfunction[21]
- Increased estrogen levels[22]
- An "Authoritarian" harm avoidance increase alongside higher serotonin and prolactin[23]
- Increased fear and anxiety[24]
- Migraines[5]
- Higher incidences of vascular disease and hypertension[25]
- Rapid decreases in blood flow to the brain[26]

Another disturbing thing to note, is that it's been found that roughly 50% of studies done showing negative effects of SSRIs go completely unpublished, due to financial conflicts of interest between drug companies and the medical journals.[27-28]

In cases of overdoses on SSRIs and 5-HTP supplements, people experience symptoms of "serotonin syndrome," with tremors, seizures, and heart failure. The antidote is antiserotonin drugs, which will save the patient's life.

Organs in the body, such as the liver and the lungs, actually have innate defense enzymes, such as indoleamine 2,3-dioxygenase, that are designed to destroy excess serotonin. However, in order for these enzymes to mobilize against serotonin properly, adequate carbon dioxide needs to be present, therefore the glucose metabolism is vital for lowering serotonin.

PUFA consumption encourages the conversion of L-tryptophan into serotonin, one of the many reasons I recommend avoiding dietary PUFAs.

The most common symptoms of excess serotonin are high blood pressure, gut problems & intestinal irritation, gynecomastia (in men), aggressiveness, insomnia, low testosterone, low thyroid hormones, liver dysfunction, high stress hormone levels, depression, anxiety, sore muscles or joints, behavioral passivity & harm avoidance, lack of creativity, hair loss, fat gain, low energy levels… all symptoms of hypothyroidism in general. Everything is connected in your body.

Patterns present themselves, and we need to pay close attention to them.

For lowering excess serotonin levels quickly and naturally, I recommend the following natural supplements:

1. Vitamin B3 (as niacinamide)
2. Theanine[29-30]
3. BCAAs
4. Amino acids such as glycine and proline (rich in collagen

and bone broth)
5. Activated charcoal
6. Mucuna Pruriens (standardized at 15% L-DOPA)

And for alleviating depression symptoms, I recommend also considering:

1. Vitamin B9 (as folate)
2. Magnesium (glycinate, citrate, or aspartate)

I also recommend that you get a full micronutrient analysis to identify deficiencies, since the deficiencies are actually what causes depression symptoms in the first place. Test for heavy metal levels in your blood as well, especially copper.

The Thermo Diet food guidelines in the next chapter of this book, like eating raw carrots, are inherently designed to properly regulate excess serotonin in your body, so please refer to those resources for nutrition suggestions.

CHAPTER TEN

HOW TO EAT THERMO

THE THERMO FOOD PYRAMID

Alright now, this is where the rubber meets the road.

Now that you fully understand the framework within which we will be operating on Thermo, I want to take this section to fully flesh out all of the specific foods - which ones to eat and which ones to avoid - that will take Thermo from being a concept into being a real, tangible part of your life moving forward.

We will walk through carbohydrate, fat, and protein sources that fit the Thermo guidelines and, where appropriate, I will elaborate with further detail on certain choices.

One of the great things about eating Thermo is how amazingly simple it is.

Where diets fail is in their complexity, their sense of restriction, and the fact that they give the individual the sense that it is a temporary thing that they only need to do for a short period of time before reverting back to their old habits.

In those cases, people feel severely restricted and the Law of Compensation is bound to swing the pendulum back to the other side sooner or later, leaving the person feeling guilty and full of shame for "falling off the wagon" once again.

Thermo isn't like that at all.

Thermo is really just a way of life.

Because it is the optimal way for your body to get the nutrients it needs, and because you eat plenty of delicious carbohydrates, meats, and fats, your cravings will literally disappear within the first month of going Thermo.

This is an incredible advantage to aiding in lifestyle design, making this truly just 'the way you eat" instead of a short term diet. Cravings are your body's natural compensation response, usually to deficiency of some kind.

Since Thermo foods are so easily digestible, they enhance your gut health and micronutrient absorption, and they contain so many easily available vitamins and minerals without any antinutrients, it's no wonder your cravings disappear so quickly - you're giving your body all the nutrients it needs and you can actually digest them all!

To make this process as easy for my readers as possible I designed a helpful tool: the Thermo Food Pyramid.

Most countries use a food pyramid of some kind, passed down from the government to the people, prescribing what the population should eat, so everyone reading this should be familiar with the concept.

The Thermo Food Pyramid however, is a bit more nuanced, which should make it even more helpful at a glance.

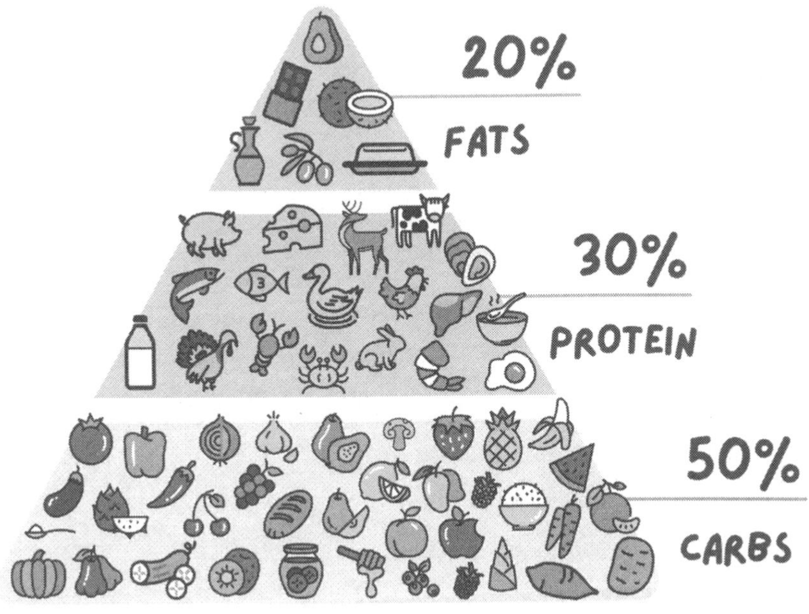

All of the foods within the pyramid are within the Thermo guidelines. However, I've added several cool new dimensions to it, namely in the form of an X and Y axis.

The X axis indicates a ratio scale, from bottom to top, of the % of macronutrient consumption relative to a 100% whole. This might sound complicated but it's super simple.

The foundation of the pyramid is the carbohydrates. This X axis scale merely demonstrates that, since carbohydrates are the foundation of the pyramid, they should be consumed in a higher proportion relative to all of the other macronutrients: fats and protein.

Protein is next up the scale, then fat. To recap, this is a simple way of seeing that carbohydrates should make up the bulk of the daily food consumption, with a moderate amount of protein, and less fat. Easy.

The other element at play on the pyramid is the Y axis which demonstrates a scale from "Less" to "More" which serves as an easy way to quickly prioritize certain sources of each level on the pyramid in your daily intake.

For example, if a food is further to the right of the pyramid, this would indicate that I recommend you to consume that food source more often than one that is further to the left of the pyramid. The factors that influence this scale include digestibility, nutrient availability, access to quality sourcing, and so forth. The foods further to the right of the food pyramid are considered the superfoods of Thermo.

Fruits and Roots!...

In this spirit of keeping things simple, I want to share a phrase that will help you remember whether or not something is Thermo.

Understand that Thermo isn't making a big restrictive list of things you can or can't eat - it's about creating a thinking framework within which you can make decisions for yourself, to make your health better.

Certain things fit within that framework, others don't. It's as simple as that.

Over the multi-year beta testing phase of the Thermo principles with the 1500 person beta test group, I also avidly shared Thermo with my friends, family, and business network. Many men and women experimented on it and had incredible results. Often people who experienced the most promising health improvements were shifting off of the keto diet over to Thermo.

One of my friends, a business owner and founder of a rather large health company local in my town of Boulder, CO named Michael summed it up as only an expert marketer like him could: Thermo is "fruits and roots!"

I love that simple way of defining it.

I would add the "meats" part to it as well, so it's "fruits, roots, and meats" but the simplicity and almost musical nature of "fruits and roots" is pretty awesome so feel free to use whichever phrase you find most helpful to remember whether something is Thermo or not.

Thermo Carbohydrates

This section is devoted to the most heavenly of macronutrients: carbs.

The characteristics of Thermo carb sources are simple: they don't contain mineral-leaching antinutrients, they're easy to digest and use for energy, and they taste incredible.

As you will see, there are nearly endless combinations of using these food sources together to create exceptional, delicious meals for you and your family that will continually support your hormonal health and metabolism.

Also, for those of you who still may have some sort of fear around consuming carbohydrates, thanks to the anti-carb movement of the past 10 years: don't worry, carbs don't make you fat.

When your body is getting fed from these nutrient-dense carb sources regularly your metabolism will steadily increase with help from your healthy thyroid gland. As long as you're not overeating, which is actually quite difficult on full Thermo nutrition, you will notice that you can eat a ton of carbohydrates and get steadily leaner and leaner over time. You will speed up your results by combining some form of regular exercise to the mix. I recommend daily walking and weight training a few times per week.

Let's look at carbs.

Fruits

Fruits form a cornerstone of your carbohydrate consumption when you're Thermo.

Fruits are an easily digestible vehicle for a rich array of vitamins and minerals alongside important prebiotic fibers that feed the probiotic bacteria strains in your gut so you can better assimilate the nutrients you're receiving.

While consuming whole fruits is preferable, since the fructose is best handled by the body alongside the naturally present fibers in the fruit itself, fresh squeezed fruit juice can also be a good option for consumption.

Choose organic fruits to lower the pesticide load.

Below is a comprehensive list of the fruits you should consume. You may notice that many of the foods on this list might be considered to be vegetables by the general public. However, this is false; they are indeed, fruits:

Fruits: (Buy Organic)

- Avocados
- Bananas
- Pineapple
- Oranges
- Watermelon
- Honeydew Melon
- Cantaloupe Melon
- Cucumbers
- Plums
- Limes
- Lemons
- Pears
- Kiwi
- Onions
- Papayas
- Mangoes
- Blueberries
- Blackberries
- Plantains
- Garlic
- Pomegranate
- Goji Berries
- Acai Berries
- Raspberries
- Mushrooms (Fungi)
- Peaches
- Pickles

- Olives
- Tomatoes
- Grapefruits
- Nectarines
- Apples
- Bell peppers
- Chilis
- Grapes
- Cherries
- Strawberries
- Pumpkin (Not Seeds Just Flesh)

Starches

Specific starch sources will likely form another cornerstone of your Thermo diet.

The important thing about starch selection is that, with a grain like rice for example, you choose white rice over brown rice.

The idea that brown rice is healthier than white rice for you is not just a myth, but a dangerous myth that is actively harming the health of millions of people.

I know we've all heard the incessant parroting in recent decades about brown rice being a healthy option. But, for some reason, it seems that all mainstream advice, especially in the health arena, is the inverse of the truth.

In fact, the more philosophically inclined of us might be ready to point out that life seems to be a steady process of waking up to the fact that much of what you've believed since birth has turned out to be a lie, where the world you were born into is built upon beliefs that are quite simply inversions of Truth.

The great philosopher Baltasar Gracian put it simply… "Life's greatest trick is that we are born asleep, and die awake." Though, admittedly 99% of humanity likely dies asleep.

That is why it's paramount for us to stop making assumptions, do not hold anything as a fact until you thoroughly examine it, especially when you hear the echo chamber of the unthinking masses repeating said dogma. That's when you should REALLY question it.

Every single thing you put into your body either brings you closer to perfect health, or further away from it.

I refer to these things as activators, and blockers respectively.

And I refer to that state of perfect health as "Thermo." We are born in arguably the most perfect state of health we will ever be in, barring prenatal developmental issues. Our skin is soft and glowing, we have boundless energy, sleep soundly, endless curiosity and imagination with a limitless capacity for rapid learning. The plasticity of our brain is incredible when we are young and still in Thermo. But over the years, the decades, we introduce more and more blockers into our bodies. Substances like certain foods and endocrine disrupting chemicals, that pull our bodies away from Thermo, away from perfect health.

My mission is to help you get back to Thermo. To put yourself back on the path to that endless energy and vitality once again.

Where did the Brown Rice Myth come from?

You may remember, back in the early 2000's when the "Whole Grain" health fad started blowing up.

It seemed like you couldn't walk into any grocery store without seeing the words Whole Grain plastered all over the package and label. Book stores were packed with new diet guru books proclaiming the health benefits of Whole Grains, and you couldn't turn on daytime television without either seeing talk and morning shows doing segments on Whole Grains or seeing commercials for cereals, breads, and meal replacement bars singing the praises of Whole Grains.

But where did this craze even come from??

Most of us don't think about it when things like this are happening, mostly because the fad or craze is so pervasive that all the hearsay surrounding it masquerades as "common knowledge." Everyone accepts it as fact.

This is propaganda at its finest.

And for those of you who are skeptical about propaganda, just read Edward Bernays' book "Propaganda" - he invented mass control via modern propaganda as a science. Population health propaganda is an extremely common form of mass control.

It was during this time that the Brown Rice Myth was born. First, people started saying that brown rice is healthier than white rice due to the fact that it's a whole grain. Then the glycemic index started to be widely used in health marketing, further demonizing white rice vs brown rice. And now with the massive demonization of simple carbohydrates, the brainwashing seems complete. Everyone who considers themself health conscious will automatically choose brown rice over white rice.

What caused this whole grain fad to start?

The answer: The US federal government.

In 1999, the FDA issued a statement that allowed for the "FDA Approved" health claim of the following,[1]

"Diets rich in whole grain foods and other plant foods, and low in saturated fat and cholesterol, may help reduce the risk of heart disease."

Giant corporations and marketers salivate over the FDA approved health claims, mostly because the masses of sheeple trust the FDA as a health authority. Why? Because they're told to, and the government trains us to bend at the knee from the time we're children in public schools.

If the FDA approves it, it must be healthy... right?

How's that working out right now with opioids?

So when the FDA issued the statement in 1999, every major "Big Food" corporation jumped all over it - especially General Mills, the company who lobbied them for the claim - and within a year every single grocery store in the US was saturated with whole grains. The TVs and bookstores positioned all the marketing. And the masses of the general public took the bait, hook line and sinker.

But you're probably still wondering, "well, why is this a big deal? What makes brown rice unhealthy anyways?"

It can always be traced back to poisoning the general public with three things:

1. Heavy metals
2. PUFAs
3. Endocrine disrupting chemicals

And brown rice does all three.

PHYTIC ACID

First, brown rice is extremely high in a substance known as

phytic acid. All of the phytic acid is found in the bran hull, the non-digestible outer layer of the rice grain. Since white rice is characterized by the absence of the outer layer, white rice does not contain any phytic acid.

Phytic acid is a highly potent anti-nutrient. It binds minerals in your body and leeches them out of your system. Anything that contributes to the widespread micronutrient deficiency epidemic is toxic and should be avoided like the plague.

Phytic acid is a negatively charged ion at a broad pH range, and therefore chelates positively charged, vitally important minerals, such as iron, zinc, magnesium, manganese, and copper. These chelates are insoluble, making them completely unavailable to the body.[2]

Phytic acid also reduces the availability of key amino acids, namely anti-stress amino acids. In fact, many researchers consider phytic acid in the diet to be the key driver of micronutrient deficiencies, outside of actual lack of nutrient intake.[3]

Soaking the rice is also not sufficient in removing the phytic acid from the hull. The only way to get rid of the phytic acid in rice is to shuck the outer layer. Asian populations for many centuries have consumed white rice, and before machinery was available, would bring the rice through an extensive process to remove the hull. In Japan, for example, highly polished white rice was considered the food of the Kings, the rich, and the elite. Brown rice was left for the peasants.

So to sum this point up, The phytic acid in rice is only present in the bran. White rice doesn't have it. The bran is also filled with easily-oxidized PUFA oils. Also not present in white rice, which we're going to discuss now.

PUFAs

The outer layer of rice is rich in polyunsaturated fatty acids, making brown rice a toxic food for several reasons, which I'll explain here. I've talked at length about toxic PUFAs in my books, and in many articles and videos, however I'll quickly recap the main points here again for you.

First, PUFAs cause hormonal imbalance.

The most well understood effect of PUFAs on hormonal imbalance is their interference with the function of the thyroid gland. PUFAs block thyroid hormone secretion, its movement in the circulatory system, and the response of tissues to the hormone. When the thyroid hormone is deficient, the body becomes exposed to increased levels of estrogen. The thyroid hormone is essential for making the "protective hormones" progesterone and pregnenolone, so the production of these protective hormones drops when anything interferes with the function of the thyroid.

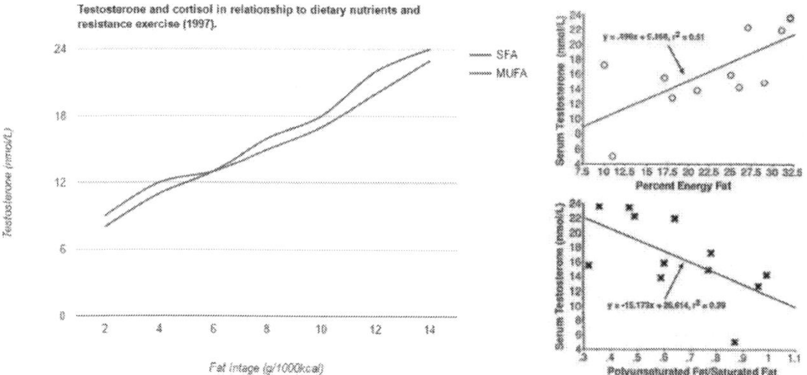

When it comes to natural steroid hormone production like testosterone, we also see a sharp drop in T production with the consumption of PUFAs.[4]

This same effect has been seen over and over again in medical research measuring hormonal impact of different types of fatty acids.[5-6]

Second, PUFAs damage the human immune system.

Vegetable oil solutions have actually been developed specifically for the purpose of knocking out the human immune system. Their effects are well documented in the medical literature,[7] and PUFAs are known to directly kill white blood cells in humans.

Vegetable oil emulsions were used in an attempt to nourish cancer patients, but it was quickly discovered that the PUFAs were suppressing their immune systems. The same products, in which vegetable oil is emulsified with water for intravenous injection, are now marketed specifically for the purpose of suppressing immunity in patients who have had organ transplants. The presence of these toxic oils in foods such as brown rice has the same harmful effect on the immune system.

Third, PUFAs cause oxidative damage.

Oxidative damage is an imbalance between the production of free radicals and the ability of the body to counteract or detoxify their harmful effects through neutralization by antioxidants.[8]

- The exposure of PUFAs to air causes the oil to go rancid; this is called oxidation, and it is the same process that occurs when oil paint "dries." Free radicals are produced in the process.
- This process is accelerated at higher temperatures, like cooking. The free radicals produced in this process react with parts of cells, such as molecules of DNA and protein and may become attached to those molecules, causing abnormalities of structure and function.

Oxidative damage in the human body leads inevitably to the cytokines triggering an inflammatory response,[8] which manifests in many different symptoms in people ranging from autoimmune disorders, to hormonal imbalances, to even more serious diseases and deficiencies such as Parkinson's, Alzheimer's, cancers and genetic mutations, chronic fatigue syndrome, atherosclerosis, heart attacks and more.

ARSENIC

In 2012 Consumer Reports released a warning against rice products due to the high levels of arsenic found in most of them, including brown rice, rice cereals, rice milks, rice cakes, crackers, and more.[10]

There was little to no arsenic found in white rice, since all of the arsenic was contained in the outer hull of the brown rice.

Where did all of this arsenic come from? And why don't people know about this? Where is the FDA and EPA on this one?

Consumer Reports specifically recommended the following:

"Our scientists are also asking regulators to prohibit agricultural practices that may lead to increases in arsenic in rice:

- *The EPA should phase out use of pesticides containing arsenic.*
- *The USDA and the EPA should end the use of arsenic-laden manure as fertilizer.*
- *The FDA should ban the feeding of arsenic-containing drugs and animal byproducts to animals."*

Dr. Chris Kresser explained the findings like this,[11]

"Brown rice, on the other hand, has significantly more arsenic than white rice and should be avoided or consumed rarely. Some of the brown rice brands tested contained at least 50% more than the safe

limit per serving, and a few even had nearly double the safe limit. Note that some of the worst offenders for arsenic are made from brown rice: processed rice products like brown rice syrup, brown rice pasta, rice cakes and brown rice crisps. These processed products are commonly consumed by those following a "healthy" whole grain rich or gluten-free diet, but they clearly pose a significant risk of arsenic overexposure, especially if a person eats more than one serving per day. Obviously, brown rice is not a food that should be a dietary staple, or even eaten on a regular basis."

The lowest levels of arsenic were found in white rice (jasmine or basmati) that was imported from other countries. Rinsing the rice (traditionally done in many cultures) further reduced the arsenic levels.

For those of you wondering what's so bad about arsenic, you might be surprised to know it's a heavy metal, and is toxic to the body at certain doses. The Center for Disease Control in the US knows very well how toxic arsenic is for the human body.

They even say on their website that Arsenic is a "confirmed human carcinogen."

Yet the USDA, FDA, and EPA continue to do nothing about the high levels of arsenic in our food supply, specifically brown rice based "whole grain" health foods. They also continue to heavily use Arsenic as a pesticide for cotton for all of our clothing.

Brown rice is a toxic food that contains high amounts of a

government admitted human carcinogen heavy metal, contains high amounts of phytic acid which is well-known to chelate vital micronutrients in the body, causing wide scale vitamin and mineral deficiencies in millions of people, and brown rice is extremely high in toxic PUFAs, which are documented in the medical literature to damage thyroid hormone production and natural reproductive hormone production, damage the immune system, and massively increase oxidative stress.

Thermo Recommended Starch Sources

So with all that out of the way, let's get to the meat and potatoes, literally.

My top recommended starch sources are tubers. Roots. Not only are they easy to digest, but they're also full of prebiotic fiber and a massively rich source of nutrients your body needs. And they taste absolutely delicious.

Below you will find a list mapping out the list of Thermo starch sources.

Starches:

- Organic Yukon Gold Potatoes
- Organic Carrots
- Organic Red Potatoes
- Organic Fingerling Potatoes

- Organic Russet Potatoes
- Organic Sweet Potatoes
- Organic Yams
- Organic Butternut Squash
- Organic Spaghetti Squash
- Organic Turnips
- Organic Beets
- Jicama
- Cassava Flour
- Coconut Flour
- Potato starch
- White Rice

Other Thermo Carbohydrate Sources

Outside of fruits and starches, there are some other carb sources that don't quite fit into those categories that are good for you to use.

Honey

First, is things like honey. Real honey is an outstanding source of vitamins and natural sugars, but it's also a good way to build the immune system against local allergens, if you can find some local honey for yourself at a farmers market.

Sourdough Bread

Bread is one of the most delicious foods that man has created.

We use it with almost every meal in regular diets around the world. So why does the Thermo philosophy say for us to not eat this?

Grains in today's society are highly contaminated with pesticides, herbicides, antifungals, and much more. If they are organic that is closer to the ideal state we want them to be in but still not quite. These grains are a massive trigger for prolactin secretion in the human body. This results in higher estrogen and stress hormones bringing us away from hormonal balance and thus the ultimate state of health we are striving to be in.

Phytic acid is a huge factor as to why we do not advocate grains as well. Phytic acid is a chelator that holds onto the minerals that it has in it. So when we see that some forms of grains, nuts, seeds, and legumes have high amounts of minerals they are not available to the body and can actually pull more out of the body as they move through it. It also deactivates trypsin which is a key enzyme for proper digestion. This leads to micronutrient deficiencies and digestive distress.

Another factor that makes grains less ideal for Thermo is the gluten content.

Gluten, especially when you are not in a good state of health, can cause massive issues in the body. Gluten is a large protein molecule found in grains. When ingested it makes its way to the intestine which is one cell thick in most areas. The large gluten molecules cause loosening of the tight junctions.

When it does this it is able to make its way into the bloodstream. Getting into the bloodstream the gluten causes an immune response in the body triggering cytokine release and thus systemic inflammation. Not only does it open the tight junctions to open up for itself but allows other large molecules to make their way through the tight junctions and cause the exact same response.

Finally if you are in a low metabolic state as defined by your waking body temperature, your resting heart rate, sleep, digestion, etc.. it is best to continue to avoid even this.

Your body is not able to handle many foods and even this can be a stressor for many. People in a low metabolic state have low stomach acid, bacterial overgrowth (in most cases), and poor peristalsis or movement of the digestive tract.

Tie all this together with really high stress levels and you have the classic case of a low metabolic state. So ensure you are mostly healthy and if not then try to stay as close to Thermo as possible by incorporating easy to digest fruit, meat, and saturated fats.

So how do we avoid this, while eating bread, and staying as Thermo as humanly possible?

1. We need to make sure that the ingredients used in the bread are organic and free of pesticides or other harmful chemicals.

2. We need to ensure the bread is additive free with as few ingredients as possible.
3. We need to ensure the grains used are fermented. This ensures the antinutrients such as phytic acid and gluten are broken down and harm free. A fermentation of 4 hours at minimum is going to allow for these to be broken down properly.
4. Make sure that it doesn't have any extra nuts, grains, seeds, soy, etc..
5. Make sure there are no additional oils used in the bread such as vegetable oils. It's very common for commercial bakers to use sunflower or safflower oil in their bread recipes. Check labels.

I am talking about sourdough bread.

It is very difficult to, however, get it from the grocery store as these varieties are not fermented for long enough duration, typically not organic, and are poor quality with lots of additives.

In order to ensure we are getting a good sourdough we either need to do one of two things.

1. Bake it ourselves
2. Get it from a good bakery.

If you bake it yourself you can either make a starter from scratch or go to a good bakery and ask for them for some.

The starter grows rapidly and they have to throw some out every now and again as they simply just get too much so this shouldn't be a problem.

If you get it from a good bakery make sure to go in and ask about the process, how they make it, what they have in it, and how often they make it. This shouldn't be a problem as you are the customer spending your hard earned dollar on their product so they should be more than happy to have a short conversation over these things. If not, go to a different bakery.

When it comes down to it quality is the most important aspect of the Thermo diet, and this is not an exception. Make sure you are getting the highest quality food you can, and this will allow for the highest quality results to take place.

Masa Harina

Masa is another addition to Thermo that allows for some additional recipe concepts and delicious meals.

Masa is a traditional Mexican cornmeal.

The production process involves a complete stripping of all of the negative aspects of the corn grain itself, like phytic acid, due to the fact that the ground corn is washed in lye, otherwise known as calcium hydroxide, which is typically derived from burnt limestone and wood ash.

During this process, also called nixtamalization - or alkaline cooking - the calcium hydroxide interacts with the corn meal in such a way as to break down the antinutrients and open up access to the natural nutrients found inside the corn. This type of corn conditioning has been done for over 3000 years according to most sources. Somehow our ancestors knew the importance of preparing it this way in order to improve the nutritional value of the corn.

The main documented benefits of the nixtamalization process are:

1. It reduces the phytic acid content of the corn[12]
2. It reduces the mycotoxin content of the corn[13]
3. It destroys the tryptophan in the corn[14]
4. It provides additional nutrients in the form of calcium, zinc, potassium, and magnesium from the preparation process[15]
5. It massively increases the niacin in the food[16]
6. By conditioning the starch, it makes it very easy to digest[17]

Thermo Fats

Consuming the right types of fats is an important part of success with Thermo.

We've talked at length regarding avoiding sources of PUFAs, however now I want to give you the recommended sources of fat you should be focusing on.

Below you will find a list of the Thermo recommended fat sources:

FATS: (Buy Organic & Grass Fed)

- Butter (Without Canola Oil)
- Coconut Oil
- Animal Fats (Produced From Game Meats)
- Ghee
- Avocados
- Coconut Manna
- Coconut Flesh
- Dark Chocolate
- Cacao Nibs
- Cacao Powder
- Cacao Butter
- Goat Cheese
- Blue Cheese
- Avocado Oil (high heat cooking)
- Olive Oil (don't cook high heats with this)

A Note About Dairy

I classify dairy as an "unsafe" food.

I don't use the term "unsafe foods" to refer to foods that you should *never* eat. **It means you need to be wary of the quality**

and the source of the foods. If you purchased them at your local grocery store, then more than likely they're unsafe.
Growing evidence shows that meat and dairy produced in western countries are not fit for human consumption. You can certainly consume these foods; you just have to acquire them from the right source.

Pay attention to the foods you eat because their source truly matters.

With that said, let's talk about dairy.

The best source for dairy is fermented dairy, which includes numerous bacterial cultures that are beneficial for the human body. Typical dairy products at your local grocery store are non-fermented, non-raw, non-organic, and heavily pasteurized. Typical grocery store milk has major blockers since the content is from cows treated with artificial growth hormones and fed an unnatural diet.

Dairy in this sense is bad for the same reason meat can be bad. It all comes down to the poor treatment of the cattle. The cows are pumped full of antibiotics, which are present in the meat and milk.

Here's something else to consider: dairy cows are artificially impregnated. In the US, dairy cows are treated with estrogen so that they're constantly nursing and producing milk in an unnatural state. When mothers give birth, they naturally produce a lot of milk so the baby can feed. In industrial farms, dairy cows are constantly given estrogen so they consistently produce milk.

The problem here is that the estrogen is also in the milk, which means consumers end up drinking the estrogen. This leads to serious hormonal disruption. You do not want to be consuming estrogen in milk, and you shouldn't be giving it to your children either.

Estrogen in milk is one of the main blockers that keeps us out of a Thermo State.

Most of you reading this probably grew up drinking a glass of milk every morning or consume it with your cereal. The milk most likely came from estrogen-treated cows. Over time, this leads to inflammation and disease in consumers. This is the accumulative effects of the estrogen, antibiotics, and synthetic growth hormones.

So, what do I recommend?

If you consume dairy, then absolutely know where the product came from. Shop at your local farmer's market and talk to the suppliers to enquire about how their dairy cows are treated. New laws have also imposed new labeling requirements. Organic super markets usually carry products that lay out in detail how the ingredients are derived.

As a general rule, if the product does not specify that it's free of artificial hormones, then it probably contains all the harmful hormones we mentioned.

Thermo Proteins

Protein is made up of amino acids. Different amino acid profiles have different effects on the body. I'm going to emphasize several key amino acids here that you should be getting more of in your diet.

There is an interesting study where mice fed a high fat and high sugar diet became obese. The protein the mice consumed was derived from chicken, cod, and crab. However, another group of mice given scallop protein did not develop obesity, despite also being administered a high fat and sugar diet. What the researchers discovered was that the protein in scallops had a different amino acid profile compared to chicken, cod, and crab.

The scallop protein was high in two specific amino acids: glycine and taurine.

Glycine

I've talked about glycine and taurine at lengths in prior content. Both are essential for hormonal health. The Thermo Diet protocol recommends eating more glycine-rich protein. Gelatin is one terrific source, though you can also take a glycine supplement. Glycine stimulates an anti-stress hormonal response; it's also pro-metabolic.

Unfortunately, most meats do not contain especially high amounts of glycine. While gelatin and scallops are terrific sources, they are not exactly a modern staple in most western diets. With the Thermo Diet, you would consume these foods along with bone broth and collagen, all of which are extremely rich in glycine. Bone broth contains gelatin and collagen, both of which contain rich concentrations of glycine.

Option B is to acquire the amino acid glycine through supplementation. Multiple studies show that glycine fights against inflammation. It also protects the body against metabolic syndrome, cancer, diabetes, endotoxin release, and intestinal damage from high toxicity. Another study showed that a glycine-rich diet prolonged the lifespan of rats by 28%. Other research showed that glycine may reverse metabolic syndrome in certain rodents.

Glycine increases energy metabolism and its flow, which is a crucial element for the Thermo Diet. It also increases insulin sensitivity and decreases oxidative stress levels in humans.

Remember, glycine is an anti-stress amino acid. Foods like white rice actually contain a decent ratio of glycine to methionine. I recommend white rice without a high arsenic level. The glycine to methionine ratio is actually more impressive than that of most meats. Various researches have discovered benefits of this amino acid ratio. This includes decreased stress, increased lifespan, and obesity prevention.

Most meats and dairy contain a higher methionine to glycine ratio. On the other hand, if you're consuming the full animal, such as using its skin and bones to make broth, then you're getting a good heaping of collagen and gelatin. If you're just consuming the meat, as most people are, then you're hardly getting any glycine.

Taurine

Taurine is another important amino acid. This has been shown to protect against metabolic syndrome, livery injury, and brain damage. Taurine intake is actually quite high in a traditional Japanese diet. Some people attribute this to the demographic's longevity.

Supplementing about 1.5 to six grams of taurine daily has been shown to protect the body against metabolic syndrome, liver disease, and the effects of chemotherapy. As you can see, this is a very promising amino acid.

If you're not already consuming a lot of glycine and taurine, then I highly recommend you do so.

You can eat more foods like shellfish or get them through supplementation. These amino acids are far more beneficial than the amino acids found in, say, a chicken breast or lean steak. This runs contrary to what you may hear from bodybuilders and others in the fitness niche.

Thermo Protein Sources:

With that in mind, please follow these protein source recommendations in order to get the best results from your journey following the Thermo Diet.

PROTEINS: Meats: (Buy Organic & Grass Fed)

- Wild game meats
- Venison
- Turkey
- Bison
- Elk
- Axis Wild Boar
- Grass Fed Free Range Beef
- Eggs
- Collagen
- Bone Broth
- Gelatin
- Liver
- Kidneys
- Shrimp
- Oysters
- Squid
- Sole
- Cod
- Crab

- Scallops
- Orange Roughy
- Mahi Mahi
- Pollock
- Lobster
- Halibut
- Scallops
- Rockfish
- Flounder
- Sushi Grade Tuna
- Chicken (free range organic)

Thermo Approved Plant Proteins

One of the best things that comes with adopting the Thermo lifestyle and philosophies is the ethical aspect that comes with it. By not supporting conventional methods of farming but rather supporting pasture raised hormone and antibiotic-free practices among farmers the animals are allowed to live lives the way they were meant to up until the time of slaughter.

However, this can still be very controversial among many people who are avoiding animal products for ethical reasons. This is perfectly okay, although from a non-biased hormonal and metabolic perspective it is not ideal as animal meat and animal products are rich in B vitamins, zinc, carnitine, saturated fat, copper, phosphorus, and iron (only when and if deficient).

As a plant-based Thermo follower, taking a micronutrient test is going to be key in optimizing your health.

Making sure you are not deficient in anything and supplementing with a good amount of the essential vitamins and minerals that are difficult to get in plants is going to be ideal and is going to help you maximize your health on all levels.

One thing that we have seen in the Thermo community is that the people who are plant-based are having trouble getting their minimum requirement of protein (which is around .6-.65 grams per pound of bodyweight) because there are not that many plant sourced proteins that are Thermo approved.

However, hopefully the suggestions following will help you get that protein and keep you completely plant based if that is your choice.

The biggest thing that you're going to want to pay attention to when looking to purchase a good plant based protein is the absence of estrogenic compounds like isoflavones, phytoestrogens and PUFAs.

The main sources to avoid are flax, soy, nuts and seeds. I highly suggest supplementing with a few things to mitigate any potential anti-nutrient effects of these protein sources.

The first is going to be vitamin E (at least 400 mg) to ensure that if there are any PUFAs in the plant-based protein source, the oxidation is limited.

Also ensure that your saturated fat intake is optimal through coconut oil, dark chocolate (free of lecithin), and cocoa butter. The best thing to look for when utilizing these plant-based protein sources is going to ensure they are as low fat as possible so that they are relatively free of PUFAs, and trying to find them fermented.

The reason you want them to be fermented is because many of these have the anti-nutrient phytic acid in them which is a chelator that attaches to minerals in the plant as well as the digestive system and makes them pass out of the body.

Allowing these sources to ferment drastically decreases the phytic acid content and allows for the nutrients within them to become more available for the body to absorb.

Hemp protein is a great source of protein, if you can find it fermented it is going to be ideal, with as little fat as possible.

Fermented Pea protein is a complete protein. Make sure it is consumed with a Vitamin C source.

Mycoprotein, otherwise known as mushroom protein can be a complete protein depending on the type of mushroom you are consuming. This protein source is relatively hard to find for a lower price as it is usually made for a specific purpose like increased cognition.

Spirulina protein is a good source of protein but isn't as ideal as our oceans are highly polluted and can contain some toxins so making sure it is relatively fat free and organic is going to be the best option.

Potato protein is a very good source of protein and is most likely the most Thermo source of protein on this list. For every 100 grams there is upwards of 93 grams of protein from a potato protein isolate and is really low in calories.

How To Construct A Thermo Diet Nutrition Regimen

Micronutrient deficiencies are the most prevalent challenges that face the society of people that lives today. Poor farming practices deplete the soil of nutrients leading to less nutrient dense food over time. Common diets that prioritize convenience over health lead to depletion of many different nutrients in the body. Prioritizing nutrient density and health in your food will allow you to get several things.

1. Limitless Energy - By constructing a diet that is nutrient dense and eliminates nutrient deficiencies and other blockers of energy flow your cells will be able to function at their full capacity. This will lead to more energy production and allow you to feel endless energy and focus each and every single day.

2. Increased Brain Performance - Brain fog is an epidemic, ravaging the lives of people around the world. The brain is the

most metabolically active organ we have. Because of this it has one of the largest needs for nutrients. If we lack any of the nutrients it needs then it will not work properly leading to brain fog.

3. Enhanced Immune System - Immunity to the diseases and illnesses that haunt this world is extremely important. Micronutrients are the weapons the immune system needs in order to fight off these ailments. Without them, the immune system is defenseless and allows the body to be attacked and taken over.

4. Decreased Rate of Aging - Chronological age is the number we say when we are asked how old we are. Biological age is the age at which your body is at. Some people can be thirty years old but have a biological age of twenty years old. If the body has an abundance of micronutrients the biological aging process can be slowed down and even reversed.

5. Fat Loss - One of the reasons that we store fat, especially in the society that exists today is because of the lack of nutrients and excess stress on the system. Micronutrient deficiencies mimic starvation internally in the human body. This results in the storage of fat because the body does not know if it is going to be able to survive without being fed properly. By correcting this and giving the body an abundance of nutrients we can train the body to be in a constant state of abundance and not have a reason to store fat in the first place.

This also allows for fat gain to take more time and fat loss to become much easier and take far less time.

Ok this all sounds awesome so how do we do it?

First and foremost the diet has to be balanced. Without a balanced diet the body will not function optimally. Eliminating macronutrients leads to micronutrient deficiencies and hormonal imbalances which does the exact opposite of what we want to do.

Moderate protein, moderate fat, and moderate to slightly high carbohydrates is going to allow for the most nutrient dense diet to come together.

After laying out your macronutrients you then have to know what the staples in your diet need to be.

These foods are the most micronutrient dense foods and are going to allow for you to alleviate not only the deficiencies in your body but the deficiencies in your wallet from buying useless supplements like a B-Complex.

These foods are liver, oysters, bone broth, eggs, red meat, fruits, and roots.

Liver is the most nutrient dense food on the face of the planet. It has been a delicacy in hundreds of cultures for thousands of years. There are even stories of packs of wolves taking down an animal and not a single part of the pack was allowed to touch the liver except for the alpha.

This is how prized this piece of the animals is even in different mammalian species! Liver is full of vitamin A, B Vitamins, Choline, Glycine, Zinc, and a whole host of other vitamins and minerals.

Incorporating a good four to six ounce portion of good grass fed liver one or two times weekly is going to be best. Oysters are the micronutrient treasure of the sea.

They are very dense in minerals like zinc and selenium as well as other vitamins and minerals. Having a good portion of oysters will allow for optimal replenishment of the body in the nutrients. Bone Broth is known as nature's multivitamin.

It is made by simmering the bones of animals for three to eight hours to allow for the nutrients found within the bones to come out. Full of glycine, proline, glutamine and various vitamins and minerals bone broth needs to be part of your daily diet no matter what. Eggs are one of the less contradictory foods on this list.

Eggs have all of the nutrients necessary to give life to a baby chick. Full of vitamins A, D, E, K, B vitamins, and choline eggs are a great addition to any diet. Having one to three eggs daily with the yolk relatively runny is going to be best.

Red meat is extremely nutrient dense, especially when it is

from a properly ethically raised animal. Red meat is less dense in inflammatory amino acids such as tryptophan and cysteine. Although poultry can be Thermo it is high in these inflammatory amino acids so red meat in most cases is going to be preferred.

Fish can be dense in heavy metals and can have an abundance of polyunsaturated fat if it is not of the right variety. So ensuring to get wild caught warm water white fish is best. Knowing this, getting a good quality organic, antibiotic and hormone free, grass fed red meat is ideal.

Fruits, especially citrus fruits are full of the water soluble vitamins like vitamin C that play a huge role in fighting disease, aging, and inflammation. Several portions of fruit a day is going to be ideal in achieving a diet that is as nutrient dense as possible. Roots, like potatoes, contain all of the nutrients needed to support the life of a plant. This makes them ideal to consume in a nutrient dense diet.

So what does a week of eating for nutrient density with these foods look like? Well it is going to vary depending on your current caloric needs and goals, as well as your food preferences but here are a couple of examples. These aren't exact and can change according to macronutrients; these are just examples to show you an example of weekly structure. You can manipulate your macronutrients and portions throughout the day based on the foods being eaten for that day.

Monday	1–3 cups pineapple 1–2 cups bone broth	12 oz potatoes 2 eggs + 2 egg whites	1–2 ripe bananas 10–12 oz potatoes 8–12 oz ground beef
Tuesday	1–3 cups pineapple 1–2 cups bone broth	12 oz potatoes 2 eggs + 2 egg whites	1–2 ripe bananas 10–12 oz potatoes 8–12 oz shrimp
Wednesday	1–3 cups pineapple 1–2 cups bone broth	12 oz potatoes 2 eggs + 2 egg whites	1–2 ripe bananas 10–12 oz potatoes 8–12 oz ground beef
Thursday	1–3 cups pineapple 1–2 cups bone broth	12 oz potatoes 2 eggs + 2 egg whites	1–2 ripe bananas 10–12 oz potatoes 6–10 oysters

Friday	1–3 cups pineapple 1–2 cups bone broth	12 oz potatoes 2 eggs + 2 egg whites	1–2 ripe bananas 10–12 oz potatoes 8–12 oz ground beef
Saturday	1–3 cups pineapple 1–2 cups bone broth	12 oz potatoes 2 eggs + 2 egg whites	1–2 ripe bananas 10–12 oz potatoes 4–6 oz liver
Sunday	1–3 cups pineapple 1–2 cups bone broth	12 oz potatoes 2 eggs + 2 egg whites	1–2 ripe bananas 10–12 oz potatoes 8–12 oz ground beef

Monday	4 eggs 4 oz liver 8-16 oz peppers 1-2 cups orange juice 12-16 oz potatoes	2-3 cups bone broth 2 cups blueberries 2 cups strawberries 2 bananas 2 tablespoons coconut oil 30-50 grams 70% dark chocolate
Tuesday	4 eggs 8 oz steak 8-16 oz peppers 1-2 cups orange juice 12-16 oz potatoes	2-3 cups bone broth 2 cups blueberries 2 cups strawberries 2 bananas 2 tablespoons coconut oil 30-50 grams 70% dark chocolate
Wednesday	4 eggs 6-10 oysters 8-16 oz peppers 1-2 cups orange juice 12-16 oz potatoes	2-3 cups bone broth 2 cups blueberries 2 cups strawberries 2 bananas 2 tablespoons coconut oil 30-50 grams 70% dark chocolate
Thursday	4 eggs 8 oz scallops 8-16 oz peppers 1-2 cups orange juice 12-16 oz potatoes	2-3 cups bone broth 2 cups blueberries 2 cups strawberries 2 bananas 2 tablespoons coconut oil 30-50 grams 70% dark chocolate

Friday	4 eggs 4 oz liver 8-16 oz peppers 1-2 cups orange juice 12-16 oz potatoes	2-3 cups bone broth 2 cups blueberries 2 cups strawberries 2 bananas 2 tablespoons coconut oil 30-50 grams 70% dark chocolate
Saturday	4 eggs 8 oz steak 8-16 oz peppers 1-2 cups orange juice 12-16 oz potatoes	2-3 cups bone broth 2 cups blueberries 2 cups strawberries 2 bananas 2 tablespoons coconut oil 30-50 grams 70% dark chocolate
Sunday	4 eggs 8 oz orange roughy 8-16 oz peppers 1-2 cups orange juice 12-16 oz potatoes	2-3 cups bone broth 2 cups blueberries 2 cups strawberries 2 bananas 2 tablespoons coconut oil 30-50 grams 70% dark chocolate

Non-Thermo Foods To Avoid

AVOID THESE CARBOHYDRATE SOURCES:

- Brown rice
- Rice bran
- Wheat
- Wheat bran
- Wheat germ
- Corn
- Quinoa
- Other random types of grains

AVOID THESE PROTEIN SOURCES :

- Beans
- Legumes
- Nuts Of Any Kind
- Seeds
- Soy
- Quorn
- Chickpeas
- Tempeh

AVOID THESE FAT SOURCES:

- All Vegetable Oils
- Fish Oils
- Seed Oils
- Margarine

Thermo Diet Approved Grocery List

CARBOHYDRATES:

Fruits: (Buy Organic)

- Avocados
- Bananas
- Pineapple
- Oranges
- Watermelon
- Honeydew Melon
- Cantaloupe Melon
- Cucumbers
- Plums
- Limes
- Lemons
- Pears
- Kiwi
- Onions
- Papayas
- Mangoes
- Blueberries
- Blackberries
- Plantains
- Garlic
- Pomegranate
- Goji Berries
- Acai Berries

- Raspberries
- Mushrooms (Fungi)
- Peaches
- Pickles
- Olives
- Tomatoes
- Grapefruits
- Nectarines
- Apples
- Bell peppers
- Chilis
- Grapes
- Cherries
- Strawberries
- Pumpkin (Not Seeds Just Flesh)

Starches:

- Organic Yukon Gold Potatoes
- Organic Carrots
- Organic Red Potatoes
- Organic Fingerling Potatoes
- Organic Russet Potatoes
- Organic Sweet Potatoes
- Organic Yams
- Organic Butternut Squash
- Organic Spaghetti Squash
- Organic Turnips
- Organic Beets

- Jicama
- Cassava Flour
- Coconut Flour
- Potato starch
- White Rice

FATS: (Buy Organic & Grass Fed)

- Butter (Without Canola Oil)
- Coconut Oil
- Animal Fats (Produced From Game Meats)
- Ghee
- Avocados
- Coconut Manna
- Coconut Flesh
- Dark Chocolate
- Cacao Nibs
- Cacao Powder
- Cacao Butter
- Goat Cheese
- Blue Cheese
- Avocado Oil (high heat cooking)
- Olive Oil (don't cook high heats with this)

PROTEINS: Meats: (Buy Organic & Grass Fed)

- Wild game meats
- Venison
- Turkey

- Bison
- Elk
- Axis Wild Boar
- Grass Fed Free Range Beef
- Eggs
- Collagen
- Bone Broth
- Gelatin
- Liver
- Kidneys
- Shrimp
- Oysters
- Squid
- Sole
- Cod
- Crab
- Scallops
- Orange Roughy
- Mahi Mahi
- Pollock
- Lobster
- Halibut
- Scallops
- Rockfish
- Flounder
- Sushi Grade Tuna
- Chicken (free range organic)

SPICES/CONDIMENTS: (Buy Organic)

- Ceylon Cinnamon
- Ground Cayenne
- Black Pepper
- Aztec Sea Salt
- Celtic Sea Salt
- Pink Himalayan Salt
- Black Lava Salt
- Ground Chipotle Pepper
- Sriracha Sauce
- Natural BBQ Tomato Sauces (Made With Cane Sugar, Spices, No Vegetable Oils, No Soy, No Seeds, Or Flower oils)
- Parsley
- Stevia
- Vanilla Extract
- Honey
- Raw Cane Sugar
- Coconut Sugar
- Kimchi
- Apple Cider Vinegar
- Sauerkraut
- Pickled Onions
- Shirataki Miracle Noodles
- Maple Syrup
- Coconut Aminos
- Turmeric
- Ginger

DRINKS: (Organic preferably in glass)

- Kombucha
- Coffee
- Mineral Water
- ZUUM by UMZU
- Spring Water
- Blue Agave Tequila
- Kvass Coconut Kefir
- Water
- Kefir
- Coconut Milk
- Coconut Water
- Pineapple Juice
- Pomegranate Juice
- Watermelon Juice
- Apple Juice
- Orange Juice
- Goat Milk
- Coca Cola (with raw cane sugar)
- Organic Red Wine

It's Time To Go Thermo!

Well that was quite the fun ride! Remember, it's not difficult to structure your nutrition in a manner that will optimize your metabolism and hormones while correcting your nutrient deficiencies. In fact, it's completely enjoyable. As all of your cravings subside in the first 30 days of going Thermo, this simply becomes *"just the way you eat."*

I sincerely hope the content of this book has helped you radically shift the way you think about the food you put into your body, and how your nutrition impacts your health.

Now without further ado... it's time to *Go Thermo!*

Sincerely,

Christopher Walker

References

Chapter 1 - Micronutrients

1. Adams, Kelly M., Karen C. Lindell, Martin Kohlmeier, and Steven H. Zeisel. 2006. "Status of Nutrition Education in Medical Schools." *The American Journal of Clinical Nutrition* 83 (4): 941S - 944S.
2. Adams, Kelly M., Martin Kohlmeier, and Steven H. Zeisel. 2010. "Nutrition Education in U.S. Medical Schools: Latest Update of a National Survey." *Academic Medicine: Journal of the Association of American Medical Colleges* 85 (9): 1537–42.
3. Frantz, David J., Craig Munroe, Stephen A. McClave, and Robert Martindale. 2011. "Current Perception of Nutrition Education in U.S. Medical Schools." *Current Gastroenterology Reports* 13 (4): 376–79.
4. Danek, Robin L., Kathryn L. Berlin, Gabi N. Waite, and Roy W. Geib. 2017. "Perceptions of Nutrition Education in the Current Medical School Curriculum." *Family Medicine* 49 (10): 803–6.
5. Castillo, Marigold, Ronald Feinstein, James Tsang, and Martin Fisher. 2016. "Basic Nutrition Knowledge of Recent Medical Graduates Entering a Pediatric Residency Program." *International Journal of Adolescent Medicine and Health* 28 (4): 357–61.
6. Gramlich, Leah M., Dana Lee Olstad, Roseanne Nasser, Laki Goonewardene, Maitreyi Raman, Sheila Innis, Sonja Wicklum, et al. 2010. "Medical Students' Perceptions of Nutrition Education in Canadian Universities." *Applied*

Physiology, Nutrition, and Metabolism = Physiologie Appliquee, Nutrition et Metabolisme 35 (3): 336–43.

7. Flegal KM, Kruszon-Moran D, Carroll MD, Fryar CD, Ogden CL. Trends in obesity among adults in the United States, 2005 to 2014. *The Journal of the American Medical Association.* 2016;315(21):2284–2291.

8. Ogden C, Carroll MD, Lawman, HG, Fryar CD, Kruszon-Moran D, et al. Trends in obesity among children and adolescents in the United States, 1988- 1994 through 2013- 2014. *The Journal of the American Medical Association.* 2016;315(21):2292–2299.

9. Fryar CD, Carroll MD, Ogden CL. Prevalence of overweight, obesity, and extreme obesity among adults aged 20 and over: United States, 1960–1962 through 2011–2014. National Center for Health Statistics Data, Health E-Stats, July 2016.

10. Fryar CD, Carroll MD, Ogden CL. Prevalence of overweight and obesity among children and adolescents aged 2–19 years: United States, 1963–1965 through 2013–2014. National Center for Health Statistics Data, Health E-Stats, July 2016.

11. Antognoli, Elizabeth L., Eileen L. Seeholzer, Heidi Gullett, Brigid Jackson, Samantha Smith, and Susan A. Flocke. 2017. "Primary Care Resident Training for Obesity, Nutrition, and Physical Activity Counseling: A Mixed-Methods Study." *Health Promotion Practice* 18 (5): 672–80.

12. Kushner, Robert F. 2016. "Providing Nutritional Care in the Office Practice: Teams, Tools, and Techniques." *The Medical Clinics of North America* 100 (6): 1157–68.

13. Kolasa, Kathryn M., and Katherine Rickett. 2010. "Barriers to Providing Nutrition Counseling Cited by Physicians: A Survey of Primary Care Practitioners." *Nutrition in Clinical Practice: Official Publication of the American Society for Parenteral and Enteral Nutrition* 25 (5): 502–9.
14. Devries, Stephen, James E. Dalen, David M. Eisenberg, Victoria Maizes, Dean Ornish, Arti Prasad, Victor Sierpina, Andrew T. Weil, and Walter Willett. 2014. "A Deficiency of Nutrition Education in Medical Training." *The American Journal of Medicine* 127 (9): 804–6.
15. Vetter, Marion L., Sharon J. Herring, Minisha Sood, Nirav R. Shah, and Adina L. Kalet. 2008. "What Do Resident Physicians Know about Nutrition? An Evaluation of Attitudes, Self-Perceived Proficiency and Knowledge." *Journal of the American College of Nutrition* 27 (2): 287–98.
16. Bacon, Francis. 1902. *Novum Organum*. P. F. Collier.
17. "Micronutrient: Meaning of Micronutrient by Lexico." *Lexico Dictionaries | English*, Lexico Dictionaries, www.lexico.com/definition/micronutrient.
18. Harvard Health Publishing. "Micronutrients Have Major Impact on Health." *Harvard Health*, www.health.harvard.edu/staying-healthy/micronutrients-have-major-impact-on-health.
19. Lewis, James L., et al. "Hypocalcemia (Low Level of Calcium in the Blood) - Hormonal and Metabolic Disorders." *Merck Manuals Consumer Version*, Merck Manuals, www.merckmanuals.com/home/hormonal-and-metabolic-disorders/electrolyte-balance/hypocalcemia-low-level-of-calcium-in-the-blood.

20. Begic-Karup, S., B. Wagner, W. Raber, B. Schneider, A. Hamwi, W. Waldhäusl, and H. Vierhapper. 2001. "Serum Calcium in Thyroid Disease." *Wiener Klinische Wochenschrift* 113 (1-2): 65–68.

21. Fong, Jeremy, and Aliya Khan. 2012. "Hypocalcemia: Updates in Diagnosis and Management for Primary Care." *Canadian Family Physician Medecin de Famille Canadien* 58 (2): 158–62.

22. Nordholm, Anders, Maria L. Mace, Eva Gravesen, Klaus Olgaard, and Ewa Lewin. 2015. "A Potential Kidney-Bone Axis Involved in the Rapid Minute-to-Minute Regulation of Plasma Ca2+." *BMC Nephrology* 16 (March): 29.

23. Al Raiisi, Fatma, Derek Stewart, Fernando Fernandez-Llimos, Teresa M. Salgado, Moustafa Fahmy Mohamed, and Scott Cunningham. 2019. "Clinical Pharmacy Practice in the Care of Chronic Kidney Disease Patients: A Systematic Review." *International Journal of Clinical Pharmacy* 41 (3): 630–66.

24. Duda, Johanna, Christina Pötschke, and Birgit Liss. 2016. "Converging Roles of Ion Channels, Calcium, Metabolic Stress, and Activity Pattern of Substantia Nigra Dopaminergic Neurons in Health and Parkinson's Disease." *Journal of Neurochemistry* 139 Suppl 1 (October): 156–78.

25. Cosman, F., S. J. de Beur, M. S. LeBoff, E. M. Lewiecki, B. Tanner, S. Randall, R. Lindsay, and National Osteoporosis Foundation. 2014. "Clinician's Guide to Prevention and Treatment of Osteoporosis." *Osteoporosis International: A Journal Established as Result of Cooperation between the European Foundation for Osteoporosis and the National*

Osteoporosis Foundation of the USA 25 (10): 2359–81.

26. Cizza, Giovanni, Svetlana Primma, and Gyorgy Csako. 2009. "Depression as a Risk Factor for Osteoporosis." *Trends in Endocrinology and Metabolism: TEM* 20 (8): 367–73.
27. Bröer, Stefan, and Angelika Bröer. 2017. "Amino Acid Homeostasis and Signalling in Mammalian Cells and Organisms." *Biochemical Journal* 474 (12): 1935–63.
28. National Research Council (US) Subcommittee on the Tenth Edition of the Recommended Dietary Allowances. 1989. *Protein and Amino Acids*. National Academies Press (US).
29. Hou, Yongqing, Yulong Yin, and Guoyao Wu. 2015. "Dietary Essentiality of 'Nutritionally Non-Essential Amino Acids' for Animals and Humans." *Experimental Biology and Medicine* 240 (8): 997–1007.
30. Meijer, Alfred J., Séverine Lorin, Edward F. Blommaart, and Patrice Codogno. 2015. "Regulation of Autophagy by Amino Acids and MTOR-Dependent Signal Transduction." *Amino Acids* 47 (10): 2037–63.
31. Bender, David A. 2003. *Nutritional Biochemistry of the Vitamins*. Cambridge University Press.
32. O'Mahony, S. M., G. Clarke, Y. E. Borre, T. G. Dinan, and J. F. Cryan. 2015. "Serotonin, Tryptophan Metabolism and the Brain-Gut-Microbiome Axis." *Behavioural Brain Research* 277 (January): 32–48.
33. Keszthelyi, D., F. J. Troost, and A. A. M. Masclee. 2009. "Understanding the Role of Tryptophan and Serotonin Metabolism in Gastrointestinal Function." *Neurogastroenterology and Motility: The Official Journal of the*

European Gastrointestinal Motility Society 21 (12): 1239–49.

34. Xiao, Tong, Cheri M. Ackerman, Elizabeth C. Carroll, Shang Jia, Adam Hoagland, Jefferson Chan, Bao Thai, Christine S. Liu, Ehud Y. Isacoff, and Christopher J. Chang. 2018. "Copper Regulates Rest-Activity Cycles through the Locus Coeruleus-Norepinephrine System." *Nature Chemical Biology* 14 (7): 655–63.
35. Williams, R. C., D. R. Baker, and J. A. Schmit. 1973. "Analysis of Water-Soluble Vitamins by High-Speed Ion-Exchange Chromatography." *Journal of Chromatographic Science* 11 (12): 618–24.
36. DeLuca, H. 2012. *The Fat-Soluble Vitamins*. Springer Science & Business Media.
37. Ammerman, Clarence B., David P. Baker, and Austin J. Lewis. 1995. *Bioavailability of Nutrients for Animals: Amino Acids, Minerals, Vitamins*. Elsevier.
38. Rucker, Robert B., Andrea J. Fascetti, and Carl L. Keen. 2008. "Trace Minerals." In *Clinical Biochemistry of Domestic Animals*, 663–93. Elsevier.
39. Castillo-Durán, C., and F. Cassorla. 1999. "Trace Minerals in Human Growth and Development." *Journal of Pediatric Endocrinology & Metabolism: JPEM* 12 (5 Suppl 2): 589–601.
40. Milner, J. A. 1990. "Trace Minerals in the Nutrition of Children." *The Journal of Pediatrics* 117 (2 Pt 2): S147–55.
41. Mc Dowell, Lee R., Nancy Wilkinson, Rachel Madison, and Tara Felix. n.d. "Vitamins and Minerals Functioning as Antioxidants with Supplementation Considerations." https://animal.ifas.ufl.edu/apps/dairymedia/RNS/2007/McDowell.pdf.

42. Pitzer, Kenneth S., and Janice J. Kim. 1993. "Thermodynamics of Electrolytes.: IV. Activity and Osmotic Coefficients for Mixed Electrolytes." In *Molecular Structure and Statistical Thermodynamics*, 1:413–19. World Scientific Series in 20th Century Chemistry. WORLD SCIENTIFIC.

43. "Overview of Sodium's Role in the Body - Hormonal and Metabolic Disorders - Merck Manuals Consumer Version." n.d. Merck Manuals Consumer Version. Merck Manuals. Accessed March 9, 2020. https://www.merckmanuals.com/home/hormonal-and-metabolic-disorders/electrolyte-balance/overview-of-sodium-s-role-in-the-body?query=sodium.

44. "Overview of Potassium's Role in the Body - Hormonal and Metabolic Disorders - Merck Manuals Consumer Version." n.d. Merck Manuals Consumer Version. Merck Manuals. Accessed March 9, 2020. https://www.merckmanuals.com/home/hormonal-and-metabolic-disorders/electrolyte-balance/overview-of-potassium-s-role-in-the-body?query=potassium.

45. "Overview of Calcium's Role in the Body - Hormonal and Metabolic Disorders - Merck Manuals Consumer Version." n.d. Merck Manuals Consumer Version. Merck Manuals. Accessed March 9, 2020. https://www.merckmanuals.com/home/hormonal-and-metabolic-disorders/electrolyte-balance/overview-of-calcium-s-role-in-the-body?query=calcium.

46. "Overview of Magnesium's Role in the Body - Hormonal and Metabolic Disorders - Merck Manuals Consumer Version." n.d. Merck Manuals Consumer Version.

Merck Manuals. Accessed March 9, 2020. https://www.merckmanuals.com/home/hormonal-and-metabolic-disorders/electrolyte-balance/overview-of-magnesium-s-role-in-the-body?query=magnesium.

47. "Overview of Phosphate's Role in the Body - Hormonal and Metabolic Disorders - Merck Manuals Consumer Version." n.d. Merck Manuals Consumer Version. Merck Manuals. Accessed March 9, 2020. https://www.merckmanuals.com/home/hormonal-and-metabolic-disorders/electrolyte-balance/overview-of-phosphate-s-role-in-the-body.

48. "Micronutrient Deficiency - an Overview | ScienceDirect Topics." n.d. Accessed March 9, 2020. https://www.sciencedirect.com/topics/agricultural-and-biological-sciences/micronutrient-deficiency.

49. CDC. 2020. "Micronutrient Facts." Centers for Disease Control and Prevention. March 4, 2020. https://www.cdc.gov/nutrition/micronutrient-malnutrition/micronutrients/index.html.

50. Progress, Current, and Iron Deficiencies. n.d. "The Micronutrient Report." https://www.nutritionintl.org/content/user_files/2017/06/The-Micronutrient-Report-Current-Progress-and-Trends-in-the-Control-of-Vitamin-A-Iodine-and-Iron-Deficiencies.pdf.

51. "Global, regional, and national trends in haemoglobin concentration and prevalence of total and severe anaemia in children and pregnant and non-pregnant women for 1995-2011: a systematic analysis of population-representative data." n.d. Accessed March 9, 2020. https://doi.org/10.1016/

S2214-109X(13)70001-9.

52. Remely, Marlene, Barbara Stefanska, Luca Lovrecic, Ulrich Magnet, and Alexander G. Haslberger. 2015. "Nutriepigenomics: The Role of Nutrition in Epigenetic Control of Human Diseases." *Current Opinion in Clinical Nutrition and Metabolic Care* 18 (4): 328–33.

53. Skeaff, Sheila A. 2011. "Iodine Deficiency in Pregnancy: The Effect on Neurodevelopment in the Child." *Nutrients* 3 (2): 265–73.

54. "Sustainable Elimination Of Iodine Deficiency." Unicef. https://www.unicef.org/publications/files/Sustainable_Elimination_of_Iodine_Deficiency.pdf.

55. Zimmermann, Michael B. 2009. "Iodine Deficiency." *Endocrine Reviews* 30 (4): 376–408.

56. "nutrition_report_2013.pdf." Unicef. https://www.unicef.org/media/files/nutrition_report_2013.pdf.

57. "WHO | Vitamin A Supplementation for Infants and Children 6–59 Months of Age." 2018, July. https://www.who.int/nutrition/publications/micronutrients/guidelines/vas_6to59_months/en/.

58. Shah, Dheeraj, and H. P. S. Sachdev. n.d. "Zinc Deficiency in Pregnancy and Fetal Outcome." https://doi.org/10.1301/nr.2006.jan.15–30.

59. Molloy, Anne M., Peadar N. Kirke, Lawrence C. Brody, John M. Scott, and James L. Mills. 2008. "Effects of Folate and Vitamin B12 Deficiencies during Pregnancy on Fetal, Infant, and Child Development." *Food and Nutrition Bulletin* 29 (2 Suppl): S101–11; discussion S112–15.

60. Sakuyama, Hiroe, Minami Katoh, Honoka Wakabayashi,

Anthony Zulli, Peter Kruzliak, and Yoshio Uehara. 2016. "Influence of Gestational Salt Restriction in Fetal Growth and in Development of Diseases in Adulthood." *Journal of Biomedical Science* 23 (January): 12.

61. Mineral Resources International. 2019. "Significant Risks of Low Magnesium During Pregnancy | Mineral Resources International Inc." Mineral Resources International Inc. May 15, 2019. https://www.mineralresourcesint.com/low-magnesium-during-pregnancy/.

62. Mahadevan, Shriraam, V. Kumaravel, and R. Bharath. 2012. "Calcium and Bone Disorders in Pregnancy." *Indian Journal of Endocrinology and Metabolism* 16 (3): 358–63.

63. Khayat, Samira, Hamed Fanaei, and Abdolhakim Ghanbarzehi. 2017. "Minerals in Pregnancy and Lactation: A Review Article." *Journal of Clinical and Diagnostic Research: JCDR* 11 (9): QE01–05.

64. Varsi, Kristin, Bjørn Bolann, Ingrid Torsvik, Tina Constanse Rosvold Eik, Paul Johan Høl, and Anne-Lise Bjørke-Monsen. 2017. "Impact of Maternal Selenium Status on Infant Outcome during the First 6 Months of Life." *Nutrients* 9 (5). https://doi.org/10.3390/nu9050486.

65. Ezzati, Majid, Alan D. Lopez, Anthony Rodgers, Stephen Vander Hoorn, Christopher J. L. Murray, and Comparative Risk Assessment Collaborating Group. 2002. "Selected Major Risk Factors and Global and Regional Burden of Disease." *The Lancet* 360 (9343): 1347–60.

66. Caulfield, Laura E., Stephanie A. Richard, Juan A. Rivera, Philip Musgrove, and Robert E. Black. 2011. "Stunting, Wasting, and Micronutrient Deficiency Disorders." *In Disease*

Control Priorities in Developing Countries, edited by Dean T. Jamison, Joel G. Breman, Anthony R. Measham, George Alleyne, Mariam Claeson, David B. Evans, Prabhat Jha, Anne Mills, and Philip Musgrove. Washington (DC): World Bank.

67. Bhan, M. K., H. Sommerfelt, and T. Strand. 2001. "Micronutrient Deficiency in Children." *The British Journal of Nutrition* 85 Suppl 2 (May): S199–203.

68. Shenkin, A. 2006. "Micronutrients in Health and Disease." *Postgraduate Medical Journal* 82 (971): 559–67.

69. Saklayen, Mohammad G. 2018. "The Global Epidemic of the Metabolic Syndrome." *Current Hypertension Reports* 20 (2): 12.

70. "General Information/Press Room | American Thyroid Association." n.d. American Thyroid Association. Accessed March 9, 2020. https://www.thyroid.org/media-main/press-room/.

71. Dunn, Donna, and Carla Turner. 2016. "Hypothyroidism in Women." *Nursing for Women's Health* 20 (1): 93–98.

72. Calton, Jayson B. 2010. "Prevalence of Micronutrient Deficiency in Popular Diet Plans." *Journal of the International Society of Sports Nutrition* 7 (June): 24.

73. Akande, K. E., U. D. Doma, H. O. Agu, and H. M. Adamu. 2010. "Major Antinutrients Found in Plant Protein Sources: Their Effect on Nutrition." *Pakistan Journal of Nutrition* 9 (8): 827–32.

74. Lopez, H. Walter, Fanny Leenhardt, Charles Coudray, and Christian Remesy. 2002. "Minerals and Phytic Acid Interactions: Is It a Real Problem for Human Nutrition?" *International Journal of Food Science & Technology* 37 (7):

727–39.

75. Masum Akond, A. S. M. Golam, Heath Crawford, Janelle Berthold, Zahirul I. Talukder, and Khwaja Hossain. 2011. "Minerals (Zn, Fe, Ca and Mg) and Antinutrient (Phytic Acid) Constituents in Common Bean." *American Journal of Food Technology* 6 (3): 235–43.

76. Gibson, Rosalind S., Karl B. Bailey, Michelle Gibbs, and Elaine L. Ferguson. 2010. "A Review of Phytate, Iron, Zinc, and Calcium Concentrations in Plant-Based Complementary Foods Used in Low-Income Countries and Implications for Bioavailability." *Food and Nutrition Bulletin* 31 (2 Suppl): S134–46.

77. Powell, J. J., R. Jugdaohsingh, and R. P. Thompson. 1999. "The Regulation of Mineral Absorption in the Gastrointestinal Tract." *The Proceedings of the Nutrition Society* 58 (1): 147–53.

78. Evans, W. J., and C. J. Martin. 1988. "Interactions of Mg(II), Co(II), Ni(II), and Zn(II) with Phytic Acid. VIII. A Calorimetric Study." *Journal of Inorganic Biochemistry* 32 (4): 259–68.

79. Zimmermann, Michael B., and Richard F. Hurrell. 2007. "Nutritional Iron Deficiency." *The Lancet* 370 (9586): 511–20.

80. Yadav, Alok Kumar, Preeti Sirohi, Saurabh Saraswat, Manjoo Rani, Manish Pratap Singh, Sameer Srivastava, and Nand K. Singh. 2018. "Inhibitory Mechanism on Combination of Phytic Acid with Methanolic Seed Extract of Syzygium Cumini and Sodium Chloride over Bacillus Subtilis." *Current Microbiology* 75 (7): 849–56.

81. Bohn, Torsten, Lena Davidsson, Thomas Walczyk, and Richard F. Hurrell. 2004. "Phytic Acid Added to White-Wheat Bread Inhibits Fractional Apparent Magnesium Absorption in Humans." *The American Journal of Clinical Nutrition* 79 (3): 418–23.

82. Cheryan, M. 1980. "Phytic Acid Interactions in Food Systems." *Critical Reviews in Food Science and Nutrition* 13 (4): 297–335.

83. Cowieson, A. J., T. Acamovic, and M. R. Bedford. 2004. "The Effects of Phytase and Phytic Acid on the Loss of Endogenous Amino Acids and Minerals from Broiler Chickens." *British Poultry Science* 45 (1): 101–8.

84. Gillooly, M., T. H. Bothwell, J. D. Torrance, A. P. MacPhail, D. P. Derman, W. R. Bezwoda, W. Mills, R. W. Charlton, and F. Mayet. 1983. "The Effects of Organic Acids, Phytates and Polyphenols on the Absorption of Iron from Vegetables." *The British Journal of Nutrition* 49 (3): 331–42.

85. Hallberg, L., M. Brune, and L. Rossander. 1989. "Iron Absorption in Man: Ascorbic Acid and Dose-Dependent Inhibition by Phytate." *The American Journal of Clinical Nutrition* 49 (1): 140–44.

86. Hallberg, L., L. Rossander, and A. B. Skånberg. 1987. "Phytates and the Inhibitory Effect of Bran on Iron Absorption in Man." *The American Journal of Clinical Nutrition* 45 (5): 988–96.

87. Hansen, M., B. Sandström, and B. Lönnerdal. 1996. "The Effect of Casein Phosphopeptides on Zinc and Calcium Absorption from High Phytate Infant Diets Assessed in Rat Pups and Caco-2 Cells." *Pediatric Research* 40 (4): 547–52.

88. Lönnerdal, B., A. S. Sandberg, B. Sandström, and C. Kunz. 1989. "Inhibitory Effects of Phytic Acid and Other Inositol Phosphates on Zinc and Calcium Absorption in Suckling Rats." *The Journal of Nutrition* 119 (2): 211–14.

89. Lonnerdal, Bo. 2002. "Phytic Acid-Trace Element (Zn, Cu, Mn) Interactions." *International Journal of Food Science & Technology* 37 (7): 749–58.

90. Ma, G., Y. Li, Y. Jin, F. Zhai, F. J. Kok, and X. Yang. 2007. "Phytate Intake and Molar Ratios of Phytate to Zinc, Iron and Calcium in the Diets of People in China." *European Journal of Clinical Nutrition* 61 (3): 368–74.

91. Rukma Reddy, N., and Shridhar K. Sathe. 2001. "Food Phytates," December.

92. Sandberg, Ann-Sofie. 2002. "Bioavailability of Minerals in Legumes." *The British Journal of Nutrition* 88 Suppl 3 (December): S281–85.

93. Sandberg, Ann-Sofie, Mats Brune, Nils-Gunnar Carlsson, Leif Hallberg, Erika Skoglund, and Lena Rossander-Hulthén. 1999. "Inositol Phosphates with Different Numbers of Phosphate Groups Influence Iron Absorption in Humans." *The American Journal of Clinical Nutrition* 70 (2): 240–46.

94. Woyengo, Tofuko A., Aaron J. Cowieson, Olayiwola Adeola, and Charles M. Nyachoti. 2009. "Ileal Digestibility and Endogenous Flow of Minerals and Amino Acids: Responses to Dietary Phytic Acid in Piglets." *The British Journal of Nutrition* 102 (3): 428–33.

95. Zhou, J. R., and J. W. Erdman Jr. 1995. "Phytic Acid in Health and Disease." *Critical Reviews in Food Science and Nutrition* 35 (6): 495–508.

96. Bohn, Torsten, Lena Davidsson, Thomas Walczyk, and Richard F. Hurrell. 2004. "Phytic Acid Added to White-Wheat Bread Inhibits Fractional Apparent Magnesium Absorption in Humans." *The American Journal of Clinical Nutrition* 79 (3): 418–23.

97. Yadav, Alok Kumar, Preeti Sirohi, Saurabh Saraswat, Manjoo Rani, Manish Pratap Singh, Sameer Srivastava, and Nand K. Singh. 2018. "Inhibitory Mechanism on Combination of Phytic Acid with Methanolic Seed Extract of Syzygium Cumini and Sodium Chloride over Bacillus Subtilis." *Current Microbiology* 75 (7): 849–56.

98. Yadav, Alok Kumar, Preeti Sirohi, Saurabh Saraswat, Manjoo Rani, Manish Pratap Singh, Sameer Srivastava, and Nand K. Singh. 2018. "Inhibitory Mechanism on Combination of Phytic Acid with Methanolic Seed Extract of Syzygium Cumini and Sodium Chloride over Bacillus Subtilis." *Current Microbiology* 75 (7): 849–56.

99. Cheryan, M. 1980. "Phytic Acid Interactions in Food Systems." *Critical Reviews in Food Science and Nutrition* 13 (4): 297–335.

100. Gupta, Raj Kishor, Shivraj Singh Gangoliya, and Nand Kumar Singh. 2015. "Reduction of Phytic Acid and Enhancement of Bioavailable Micronutrients in Food Grains." *Journal of Food Science and Technology* 52 (2): 676–84.

101. Hunt, Janet R. 2003. "Bioavailability of Iron, Zinc, and Other Trace Minerals from Vegetarian Diets." *The American Journal of Clinical Nutrition* 78 (3 Suppl): 633S – 639S.

102. Singh, Madhav, and A. D. Krikorian. 1982. "Inhibition of

Trypsin Activity in Vitro by Phytate." *Journal of Agricultural and Food Chemistry* 30 (4): 799–800.

103. Knuckles, B. E., and A. A. Betschart. 1987. "Effect of Phytate and Other Myo-Inositol Phosphate Esters on α-Amylase Digestion of Starch." *Journal of Food Science* 52 (3): 719–21.

104. Khan, Argha, and Koushik Ghosh. 2013. "Phytic Acid-Induced Inhibition of Digestive Protease and α-Amylase in Three Indian Major Carps: An in Vitro Study : INHIBITION OF CARP DIGESTIVE ENZYMES BY PHYTIC ACID." *Journal of the World Aquaculture Society* 44 (6): 853–59.

105. Knuckles, B. E., D. D. Kuzmicky, and A. A. Betschart. 1985. "Effect of Phytate and Partially Hydrolyzed Phytate on in Vitro Protein Digestibility." *Journal of Food Science* 50 (4): 1080–82.

106. Thompson, L. U., C. L. Button, and D. J. Jenkins. 1987. "Phytic Acid and Calcium Affect the in Vitro Rate of Navy Bean Starch Digestion and Blood Glucose Response in Humans." *The American Journal of Clinical Nutrition* 46 (3): 467–73.

107. Ilelaboye, N. O. A., and O. O. Pikuda. 2009. "Determination of Minerals and Anti-Nutritional Factors of Some Lesser-Known Crop Seeds." *Pakistan Journal of Nutrition* 8 (10): 1652–56.

108. Kitts, W. D., A. J. Wood, E. Swierstra, and V. C. Brink. 1959. "THE ESTROGEN-LIKE SUBSTANCES IN CERTAIN LEGUMES AND GRASSES: I. THE QUANTITATIVE DETERMINATION OF SUCH SUBSTANCES IN RED CLOVER AND OATS." *Canadian Journal of Animal Science* 39 (1): 6–13.

109. D'Mello, J. P. F. 1992. "Chemical Constraints to the Use of Tropical Legumes in Animal Nutrition." *Animal Feed Science and Technology* 38 (2): 237–61.

110. "OfficeofDietarySupplements - Magnesium." NIH. Accessed March 10, 2020. https://ods.od.nih.gov/factsheets/Magnesium-HealthProfessional/.

111. Rude RK. Magnesium. In: Coates PM, Betz JM, Blackman MR, Cragg GM, Levine M, Moss J, White JD, eds. Encyclopedia of Dietary Supplements. 2nd ed. New York, NY: Informa Healthcare; 2010:527–37.

112. RudeRK.Magnesium.In:RossAC,CaballeroB,Cousins RJ, Tucker KL, Ziegler TR, eds. Modern Nutrition in Health and Disease. 11th ed. Baltimore, Mass: Lippincott Williams & Wilkins; 2012:159–75

113. Kubota, Takeshi, Yutaka Shindo, Kentaro Tokuno, Hirokazu Komatsu, Hiroto Ogawa, Susumu Kudo, Yoshiichiro Kitamura, Koji Suzuki, and Kotaro Oka. 2005. "Mitochondria Are Intracellular Magnesium Stores: Investigation by Simultaneous Fluorescent Imagings in PC12 Cells." *Biochimica et Biophysica Acta* 1744 (1): 19–28.

114. Vitale,B.Y.J.J.,M.Nakamura,andD.M.Hegsted.n.d. "THE EFFECT OF MAGNESIUM DEFICIENCY ON OXIDATIVE PHOSPHORYLATION"." https://pdfs.semanticscholar.org/c922/c4b15c1875e4d4cc947b351e54560b78812c.pdf.

115. Weber, G., M. A. Lea, H. J. Convery, and N. B. Stamm. 1967. "Regulation of Gluconeogenesis and Glycolysis: Studies of Mechanisms Controlling Enzyme Activity." *Advances in Enzyme Regulation* 5: 257–300.

116. Rosanoff, Andrea, Connie M. Weaver, and Robert K. Rude.

2012. "Suboptimal Magnesium Status in the United States: Are the Health Consequences Underestimated?" *Nutrition Reviews* 70 (3): 153–64.

117. Isao Saito, MD, PhD; Koutatsu Maruyama, PhD; Eri Eguchi, PhD; Tadahiro Kato, MD, PhD; Ryoichi Kawamura, MD, PhD; Yasunori Takata, MD, PhD; Hiroshi Onuma, MD, PhD; Haruhiko Osawa, MD, PhD; Takeshi Tanigawa, MD, PhD. "Low Heart Rate Variability and Sympathetic Dominance Modifies the Association Between Insulin Resistance and Metabolic Syndrome" Circ J doi:10.1253/circj.CJ-17-0192. https://www.jstage.jst.go.jp/article/circj/advpub/0/advpub_CJ-17-0192/_pdf.

118. Okazaki Ryo. 2018. "[Bodyweight and bone/calcium metabolism. Obesity and vitamin D.]." *Clinical calcium* 28 (7): 947–56.

119. Jafari, Tina, Elham Faghihimani, Awat Feizi, Bijan Iraj, Shaghayegh Haghjooy Javanmard, Ahmad Esmaillzadeh, Aziz A. Fallah, and Gholamreza Askari. 2016. "Effects of Vitamin D-Fortified Low Fat Yogurt on Glycemic Status, Anthropometric Indexes, Inflammation, and Bone Turnover in Diabetic Postmenopausal Women: A Randomised Controlled Clinical Trial." *Clinical Nutrition* 35 (1): 67–76.

120. Via, Michael. 2012. "The Malnutrition of Obesity: Micronutrient Deficiencies That Promote Diabetes." *ISRN Endocrinology* 2012 (March): 103472.

121. Kaidar-Person, Orit, Benjamin Person, Samuel Szomstein, and Raul J. Rosenthal. 2008. "Nutritional Deficiencies in Morbidly Obese Patients: A New Form of Malnutrition? Part A: Vitamins." *Obesity Surgery* 18 (7):

870–76.

122. Strohmayer, Erika, Michael A. Via, and Robert Yanagisawa. 2010. "Metabolic Management Following Bariatric Surgery." *The Mount Sinai Journal of Medicine, New York* 77 (5): 431–45.

123. Pittas, Anastassios G., Joseph Lau, Frank B. Hu, and Bess Dawson-Hughes. 2007. "The Role of Vitamin D and Calcium in Type 2 Diabetes. A Systematic Review and Meta-Analysis." *The Journal of Clinical Endocrinology and Metabolism* 92 (6): 2017–29.

124. Bourlon PM, Billaudel B, Faure-Dussert A. Influence of vitamin D3 deficiency and 1,25 dihydroxyvitamin D3 on de novo insulin biosynthesis in the islets of the rat endocrine pancreas. *Journal of Endocrinology.* 1999;160(1):87–95.

125. Norman AW, Frankel BJ, Heldt AM, Grodsky GM. Vitamin D deficiency inhibits pancreatic secretion of insulin. *Science.* 1980;209(4458):823–825.

126. Tanaka Y, Seino Y, Ishida M, et al. Effect of vitamin D3 on the pancreatic secretion of insulin and somatostatin. *Acta Endocrinologica.* 1984;105(4):528–533.

127. Brock KE, Huang W-Y, Fraser DR, et al. Diabetes prevalence is associated with serum 25-hydroxyvitamin D and 1,25-dihydroxyvitamin D in US middle-aged Caucasian men and women: a cross-sectional analysis within the prostate, lung, colorectal and ovarian cancer screening trial. *British Journal of Nutrition.* 2011;106(3):339–344.

128. Grimnes G, Emaus N, Joakimsen RM, et al. Baseline serum 25-hydroxyvitamin D concentrations in the Tromsø Study 1994-95 and risk of developing type 2 diabetes

mellitus during 11 years of follow-up. *Diabetic Medicine.* 2010;27(10):1107–1115.

129. Isaia G, Giorgino R, Adami S. High prevalence of hypovitaminosis D in female type 2 diabetic population. *Diabetes Care.* 2001;24(8):p. 1496.

130. Scragg R, Holdaway I, Singh V, Metcalf P, Baker J, Dryson E. Serum 25-hydroxyvitamin D3 levels decreased in impaired glucose tolerance and diabetes mellitus. *Diabetes Research and Clinical Practice.* 1995;27(3):181–188.

131. Scragg R, Sowers M, Bell C. Serum 25-hydroxyvitamin D, diabetes, and ethnicity in the Third National Health and Nutrition Examination Survey. *Diabetes Care.* 2004;27(12):2813–2818.

132. Tahrani AA, Ball A, Shepherd L, Rahim A, Jones AF, Bates A. The prevalence of vitamin D abnormalities in South Asians with type 2 diabetes mellitus in the UK. *International Journal of Clinical Practice.* 2010;64(3):351–355.

133. Behall KM, Schofield DJ, Hallfrisch JG, Kelsay JL, Reiser S. Seasonal variation in plasma glucose and hormone levels in adult men and women. *The American Journal of Clinical Nutrition.* 1984;40(6):1352–1356.

134. Ishii H, Suzuki H, Baba T, Nakamura K, Watanabe T. Seasonal variation of glycemic control in type 2 diabetic patients. *Diabetes Care.* 2001;24(8):p. 1503.

135. Pittas, Anastassios G., Joseph Lau, Frank B. Hu, and Bess Dawson-Hughes. 2007. "The Role of Vitamin D and Calcium in Type 2 Diabetes. A Systematic Review and Meta-Analysis." *The Journal of Clinical Endocrinology and Metabolism* 92 (6): 2017–29.

136. Wolden-Kirk, Heidi, Lut Overbergh, Henrik Thybo Christesen, Klaus Brusgaard, and Chantal Mathieu. 2011. "Vitamin D and Diabetes: Its Importance for Beta Cell and Immune Function." *Molecular and Cellular Endocrinology* 347 (1-2): 106-20.

137. Mitri, J., M. D. Muraru, and A. G. Pittas. 2011. "Vitamin D and Type 2 Diabetes: A Systematic Review." *European Journal of Clinical Nutrition* 65 (9): 1005-15.

138. Nagpal J, Pande JN, Bhartia A. A double-blind, randomized, placebo-controlled trial of the short-term effect of vitamin D3 supplementation on insulin sensitivity in apparently healthy, middle-aged, centrally obese men. *Diabetic Medicine*. 2009;26(1):19-27.

139. Pittas AG, Harris SS, Stark PC, Dawson-Hughes B. The effects of calcium and vitamin D supplementation on blood glucose and markers of inflammation in nondiabetic adults. *Diabetes Care*. 2007;30(4):980-986.

140. von Hurst PR, Stonehouse W, Coad J. Vitamin D supplementation reduces insulin resistance in South Asian women living in New Zealand who are insulin resistant and vitamin D deficient-a randomised, placebo-controlled trial. *British Journal of Nutrition*. 2010;103(4):549-555.

141. Effects of vitamin D and calcium supplementation on pancreatic β cell function, insulin sensitivity, and glycemia in adults at high risk of diabetes: the Calcium and Vitamin D for Diabetes Mellitus (CaDDM) randomized controlled trial. *Mitri J, Dawson-Hughes B, Hu FB, Pittas AG Am J Clin Nutr. 2011 Aug; 94(2):486-94.*

142. Daily consumption of vitamin D- or vitamin D + calcium-

fortified yogurt drink improved glycemic control in patients with type 2 diabetes: a randomized clinical trial. *Nikooyeh B, Neyestani TR, Farvid M, Alavi-Majd H, Houshiarrad A, Kalayi A, Shariatzadeh N, Gharavi A, Heravifard S, Tayebinejad N, Salekzamani S, Zahedirad M Am J Clin Nutr. 2011 Apr; 93(4):764–71.*

143. Mertz, W., and K. Schwarz. 1959. "Relation of Glucose Tolerance Factor to Impaired Intravenous Glucose Tolerance of Rats on Stock Diets." *The American Journal of Physiology* 196 (3): 614–18.

144. Schwarz, K., and W. Mertz. 1959. "Chromium(III) and the Glucose Tolerance Factor." *Archives of Biochemistry and Biophysics* 85 (November): 292–95.

145. Brown, R. O., S. Forloines-Lynn, R. E. Cross, and W. D. Heizer. 1986. "Chromium Deficiency after Long-Term Total Parenteral Nutrition." *Digestive Diseases and Sciences* 31 (6): 661–64.

146. Freund H, Atamian S, Fischer JE. Chromium deficiency during total parenteral nutrition. *Journal of the American Medical Association*. 1979;241(5):496–498.

147. Jeejeebhoy KN, Chu RC, Marliss EB, Greenberg GR, Bruce-Robertson A. Chromium deficiency, glucose intolerance, and neuropathy reversed by chromium supplementation, in a patient receiving long term total parenteral nutrition. *The American Journal of Clinical Nutrition*. 1977;30(4):531–538.

148. Via M, Scurlock C, Raikhelkar J, Di Luozzo G, Mechanick JI. Chromium infusion reverses extreme insulin resistance in a cardiothoracic ICU patient. *Nutrition in Clinical Practice*. 2008;23(3):325–328.

149. Ekmekcioglu, C., C. Prohaska, K. Pomazal, I. Steffan, G. Schernthaner, and W. Marktl. 2001. "Concentrations of Seven Trace Elements in Different Hematological Matrices in Patients with Type 2 Diabetes as Compared to Healthy Controls." *Biological Trace Element Research* 79 (3): 205–19.

150. Kazi, Tasneem Gul, Hassan Imran Afridi, Naveed Kazi, Mohammad Khan Jamali, Mohammad Bilal Arain, Nussarat Jalbani, and Ghulam Abbas Kandhro. 2008. "Copper, Chromium, Manganese, Iron, Nickel, and Zinc Levels in Biological Samples of Diabetes Mellitus Patients." *Biological Trace Element Research* 122 (1): 1–18.

151. Rajpathak, Swapnil, Eric B. Rimm, Tricia Li, J. Steven Morris, Meir J. Stampfer, Walter C. Willett, and Frank B. Hu. 2004. "Lower Toenail Chromium in Men with Diabetes and Cardiovascular Disease Compared with Healthy Men." *Diabetes Care* 27 (9): 2211–16.

152. Broadhurst, C. Leigh, and Philip Domenico. 2006. "Clinical Studies on Chromium Picolinate Supplementation in Diabetes Mellitus--a Review." *Diabetes Technology & Therapeutics* 8 (6): 677–87.

153. "FDA Approves First Qualified Health Claim for Chromium Picolinate and Risk of Type 2 Diabetes; FDA Concludes That Chromium Picolinate Is Safe." 2005. August 29, 2005. https://www.businesswire.com/news/home/20050829005447/en/FDA-Approves-Qualified-Health-Claim-Chromium-Picolinate.

154. "Thiamin." 2017. Mayo Clinic. October 25, 2017. https://www.mayoclinic.org/drugs-supplements-thiamin/art-20366430.

155. Bettendorff, Lucien, and Pierre Wins. 2009. "Thiamin Diphosphate in Biological Chemistry: New Aspects of Thiamin Metabolism, Especially Triphosphate Derivatives Acting Other than as Cofactors." *The FEBS Journal* 276 (11): 2917–25.

156. Page, G. L. J., D. Laight, and M. H. Cummings. 2011. "Thiamine Deficiency in Diabetes Mellitus and the Impact of Thiamine Replacement on Glucose Metabolism and Vascular Disease." *International Journal of Clinical Practice* 65 (6): 684–90.

157. McGuire, Shelley. 2011. "U.S. Department of Agriculture and U.S. Department of Health and Human Services, Dietary Guidelines for Americans, 2010. 7th Edition, Washington, DC: U.S. Government Printing Office, January 2011." *Advances in Nutrition* 2 (3): 293–94.

158. Lonsdale, Derrick. 2006. "A Review of the Biochemistry, Metabolism and Clinical Benefits of Thiamin(e) and Its Derivatives." *Evidence-Based Complementary and Alternative Medicine: eCAM* 3 (1): 49–59.

159. Pincus, J. H., and K. Wells. 1972. "Regional Distribution of Thiamine-Dependent Enzymes in Normal and Thiamine-Deficient Brain." *Experimental Neurology* 37 (3): 495–501.

160. Lukienko, P. I., N. G. Mel'nichenko, I. V. Zverinskii, and S. V. Zabrodskaya. 2000. "Antioxidant Properties of Thiamine." *Bulletin of Experimental Biology and Medicine* 130 (9): 874–76.

161. Ascher, E., P. V. Gade, A. Hingorani, S. Puthukkeril, S. Kallakuri, M. Scheinman, and T. Jacob. 2001. "Thiamine Reverses Hyperglycemia-Induced Dysfunction in Cultured Endothelial Cells." *Surgery* 130 (5): 851–58.

162. "General Information/Press Room | American Thyroid Association." n.d. American Thyroid Association. Accessed March 10, 2020. https://www.thyroid.org/media-main/press-room/.

163. "Hypothyroidism (Underactive Thyroid) | NIDDK." n.d. National Institute of Diabetes and Digestive and Kidney Diseases. Accessed March 10, 2020. https://www.niddk.nih.gov/health-information/endocrine-diseases/hypothyroidism.

164. Kapil, Umesh. 2007. "Health Consequences of Iodine Deficiency." *Sultan Qaboos University Medical Journal* 7 (3): 267–72.

165. "Iodine Deficiency | American Thyroid Association." n.d. American Thyroid Association. Accessed March 10, 2020. https://www.thyroid.org/iodine-deficiency/.

166. Hess, Sonja Y. 2010. "The Impact of Common Micronutrient Deficiencies on Iodine and Thyroid Metabolism: The Evidence from Human Studies." Best Practice & Research. *Clinical Endocrinology & Metabolism* 24 (1): 117–32.

167. Wolde-Gebriel, Z., C. E. West, H. Gebru, A. S. Tadesse, T. Fisseha, P. Gabre, C. Aboye, G. Ayana, and J. G. Hautvast. 1993. "Interrelationship between Vitamin A, Iodine and Iron Status in Schoolchildren in Shoa Region, Central Ethiopia." *The British Journal of Nutrition* 70 (2): 593–607.

168. Zimmermann, Michael B., and Josef Köhrle. 2002. "The Impact of Iron and Selenium Deficiencies on Iodine and Thyroid Metabolism: Biochemistry and Relevance to Public Health." *Thyroid: Official Journal of the American Thyroid*

Association 12 (10): 867–78.

169. Nishiyama, S., Y. Futagoishi-Suginohara, M. Matsukura, T. Nakamura, A. Higashi, M. Shinohara, and I. Matsuda. 1994. "Zinc Supplementation Alters Thyroid Hormone Metabolism in Disabled Patients with Zinc Deficiency." *Journal of the American College of Nutrition* 13 (1): 62–67.

170. Hess, Sonja Y. 2010. "The Impact of Common Micronutrient Deficiencies on Iodine and Thyroid Metabolism: The Evidence from Human Studies." *Best Practice & Research. Clinical Endocrinology & Metabolism* 24 (1): 117–32.

Chapter 2 - Salt

1. Wardener, H. E. de. 1999. "Salt Reduction and Cardiovascular Risk: The Anatomy of a Myth." *Journal of Human Hypertension* 13 (1): 1–4.

2. Harvard Health Publishing. n.d. "The Trouble with Excess Salt - Harvard Health." Harvard Health. Accessed March 31, 2020.https://www.health.harvard.edu/staying-healthy/the-trouble-with-excess-salt.

3. "Salt and Sodium | Nutrition.gov." n.d. Accessed March 31, 2020. https://www.nutrition.gov/topics/whats-food/salt-and-sodium.

4. Neuman, William. 2010. "Citing Hazard, New York Says Hold the Salt." *The New York Times*, January 11, 2010. https://www.nytimes.com/2010/01/11/business/11salt.html.

5. "CDC - Salt - Sodium and the Institute of Medicine." 2019. May 9, 2019. https://www.cdc.gov/salt/sodium_iom.

htm.

6. Peat, Raymond. n.d. "Salt, Energy, Metabolic Rate, and Longevity." Accessed March 31, 2020. https://raypeat.com/articles/articles/salt.shtml.
7. Gelpi, Adriane, and Joseph D. Tucker. 2015. "After Venus, Mercury: Syphilis Treatment in the UK before Salvarsan." *Sexually Transmitted Infections* 91 (1): 68.
8. Tampa, M., I. Sarbu, C. Matei, V. Benea, and S. R. Georgescu. 2014. "Brief History of Syphilis." *Journal of Medicine and Life* 7 (1): 4–10.
9. Maurage, C., M. C. Belin, M. Robert, M. Bremond, E. Autret, and J. C. Rolland. 1989. "[Rectal injury caused by a broken thermometer. Risks related to mercury]." *Archives francaises de pediatrie* 46 (4): 277–79.
10. Chauhan, Ved, Syian Srikumar, Sarah Aamer, Mirazkar D. Pandareesh, and Abha Chauhan. 2017. "Methylmercury Exposure Induces Sexual Dysfunction in Male and Female Drosophila Melanogaster." *International Journal of Environmental Research and Public Health* 14 (10). https://doi.org/10.3390/ijerph14101108.
11. Park, Jung-Duck, and Wei Zheng. 2012. "Human Exposure and Health Effects of Inorganic and Elemental Mercury." *Journal of Preventive Medicine and Public Health = Yebang Uihakhoe Chi* 45 (6): 344–52.
12. Sarikaya, Sezgin, Ozgur Karcioglu, Didem Ay, Asli Cetin, Can Aktas, and Mustafa Serinken. 2010. "Acute Mercury Poisoning: A Case Report." *BMC Emergency Medicine* 10 (March): 7.
13. Miller, Saul, Shelley Pallan, Azim S. Gangji, Dusan

Lukic, and Catherine M. Clase. 2013. "Mercury-Associated Nephrotic Syndrome: A Case Report and Systematic Review of the Literature." *American Journal of Kidney Diseases: The Official Journal of the National Kidney Foundation* 62 (1): 135–38.

14. Sartin, J. S., and H. O. Perry. 1995. "From Mercury to Malaria to Penicillin: The History of the Treatment of Syphilis at the Mayo Clinic--1916-1955." *Journal of the American Academy of Dermatology* 32 (2 Pt 1): 255–61.

15. Tan, Siang Yong, and Yvonne Tatsumura. 2015. "Alexander Fleming (1881-1955): Discoverer of Penicillin." *Singapore Medical Journal* 56 (7): 366–67.

16. Bliss, A. Richard, Jr., and Robert W. Morrison. 1933. "A Comparative Study of Two Xanthine Diuretics *." *Journal of the American Pharmaceutical Association* 22 (5): 404–10.

17. "Acetazolamide: MedlinePlus Drug Information." n.d. Accessed April 14, 2020. https://medlineplus.gov/druginfo/meds/a682756.html.

18. "Chlorothiazide: MedlinePlus Drug Information." n.d. Accessed April 14, 2020. https://medlineplus.gov/druginfo/meds/a682341.html.

19. "Furosemide: MedlinePlus Drug Information." n.d. Accessed April 14, 2020. https://medlineplus.gov/druginfo/meds/a682858.html.

20. "Ethacrynic Acid: MedlinePlus Drug Information." n.d. Accessed April 14, 2020. https://medlineplus.gov/druginfo/meds/a682857.html.

21. Roush, George C., and Domenic A. Sica. 2016. "Diuretics for Hypertension: A Review and Update." *American Journal of*

Hypertension 29 (10): 1130–37.

22. Casu, Gavino, and Pierluigi Merella. 2015. "Diuretic Therapy in Heart Failure - Current Approaches." European Cardiology 10 (1): 42–47.
23. Morrison, R. T. 1997. "Edema and Principles of Diuretic Use." *The Medical Clinics of North America* 81 (3): 689–704.
24. Wishnofsky, Max. 1964. "Use of Diuretics in the Treatment of Obesity." *JAMA: The Journal of the American Medical Association* 187 (5): 377–377.
25. Olesen, C., C. S. de Vries, N. Thrane, T. M. MacDonald, H. Larsen, H. T. Sørensen, and EuroMAP Group. 2001. "Effect of Diuretics on Fetal Growth: A Drug Effect or Confounding by Indication? Pooled Danish and Scottish Cohort Data." *British Journal of Clinical Pharmacology* 51 (2): 153–57.
26. Klemmer Philip, Grim Clarence E., and Luft Friedrich C. 2014. "Who and What Drove Walter Kempner?" *Hypertension* 64 (4): 684–88.
27. Sakuyama, Hiroe, Minami Katoh, Honoka Wakabayashi, Anthony Zulli, Peter Kruzliak, and Yoshio Uehara. 2016. "Influence of Gestational Salt Restriction in Fetal Growth and in Development of Diseases in Adulthood." *Journal of Biomedical Science* 23 (January): 12.
28. Oppelaar, Jetta J., and Liffert Vogt. 2019. "Body Fluid-Independent Effects of Dietary Salt Consumption in Chronic Kidney Disease." *Nutrients* 11 (11). https://doi.org/10.3390/nu11112779.
29. Asayama, Kei, and Yutaka Imai. 2018. "The Impact of Salt Intake during and after Pregnancy." *Hypertension Research: Official Journal of the Japanese Society of Hypertension* 41 (1):

1–5.

30. "The Long Term Effects of Advice to Cut down on Salt in Food on Deaths, Cardiovascular Disease and Blood Pressure in Adults." n.d. Accessed April 14, 2020. https://doi.org/10.1002/14651858.CD003656.pub2.

31. "Intersalt: An International Study of Electrolyte Excretion and Blood Pressure. Results for 24 Hour Urinary Sodium and Potassium Excretion. Intersalt Cooperative Research Group." 1988. *BMJ* 297 (6644): 319–28.

32. Hooper, L., C. Bartlett, G. Davey Smith, and S. Ebrahim. 2003. "Reduced Dietary Salt for Prevention of Cardiovascular Disease." *Cochrane Database of Systematic Reviews* , no. 3: CD003656.

33. Hypertension 25: 1144–1152, 1995: Low urinary sodium is associated with greater risk of myocardial infarction among treated hypertensive men. Alderman MH, Madhavan S, Cohen H, Sealey JE, Laragh JH

34. The National Health and Nutrition Examination Survey (NHANES I). Lancet 351: 781–785, 1998: Dietary sodium intake and mortality, Alderman MH, Cohen H, Madhavan S.

35. Life, the science of biology / William K. Purves, Gordon H. Orians, H. Craig Heller. 4th ed. C1995.

36. Boundless. n.d. "ATP: Adenosine Triphosphate | Boundless Biology." Accessed April 14, 2020. https://courses.lumenlearning.com/boundless-biology/chapter/atp-adenosine-triphosphate/.

37. Atchison, Douglas K., and William H. Beierwaltes. 2013. "The Influence of Extracellular and Intracellular Calcium on the Secretion of Renin." *Pflugers Archiv: European Journal of*

Physiology 465 (1): 59–69.

38. "Cation - an Overview | ScienceDirect Topics." n.d. Accessed April 14, 2020. https://www.sciencedirect.com/topics/earth-and-planetary-sciences/cation.

39. "Anion - an Overview | ScienceDirect Topics." n.d. Accessed April 14, 2020. https://www.sciencedirect.com/topics/earth-and-planetary-sciences/anion.

40. "What Is an Ion?" n.d. Accessed April 14, 2020. http://www.qrg.northwestern.edu/projects/vss/docs/propulsion/1-what-is-an-ion.html.

41. "Salt - Chemistry Encyclopedia - Water, Uses, Examples, Metal, Gas, Uses." n.d. Accessed April 14, 2020. http://www.chemistryexplained.com/Ru-Sp/Salt.html.

42. "Naming Salts (Ionic Compounds)." n.d. Accessed April 14, 2020. https://www.stolaf.edu/depts/chemistry/courses/toolkits/121/js/naming/salts.htm.

43. "Saltiness - an Overview | ScienceDirect Topics." n.d. Accessed April 14, 2020. https://www.sciencedirect.com/topics/nursing-and-health-professions/saltiness.

44. "Ocean Island Basalt - an Overview | ScienceDirect Topics." n.d. Accessed April 14, 2020. https://www.sciencedirect.com/topics/earth-and-planetary-sciences/ocean-island-basalt.

45. Manrique, Camila, Guido Lastra, Michael Gardner, and James R. Sowers. 2009. "The Renin Angiotensin Aldosterone System in Hypertension: Roles of Insulin Resistance and Oxidative Stress." *The Medical Clinics of North America* 93 (3): 569–82.

46. Remuzzi, Giuseppe, Norberto Perico, Manuel Macia, and

Piero Ruggenenti. 2005. "The Role of Renin-Angiotensin-Aldosterone System in the Progression of Chronic Kidney Disease." *Kidney International. Supplement*, no. 99 (December): S57–65.

47. Unger, Thomas, and Jun Li. 2004. "The Role of the Renin-Angiotensin-Aldosterone System in Heart Failure." *Journal of the Renin-Angiotensin-Aldosterone System: JRAAS* 5 Suppl 1 (September): S7–10.
48. Hypertens Pregnancy. 2006;25(3):143–57. Increased sympathetic activity present in early hypertensive pregnancy is not lowered by plasma volume expansion. Metsaars WP, Ganzevoort W, Karemaker JM, Rang S, Wolf H.
49. Reivich, M., A. Alavi, A. Wolf, J. Fowler, J. Russell, C. Arnett, R. R. MacGregor, C. Y. Shiue, H. Atkins, and A. Anand. 1985. "Glucose Metabolic Rate Kinetic Model Parameter Determination in Humans: The Lumped Constants and Rate Constants for [18F]fluorodeoxyglucose and [11C] deoxyglucose." *Journal of Cerebral Blood Flow and Metabolism: Official Journal of the International Society of Cerebral Blood Flow and Metabolism* 5 (2): 179–92.
50. Boden, Guenther. 2008. "Obesity and Free Fatty Acids." *Endocrinology and Metabolism Clinics of North America* 37 (3): 635–46, viii – ix.
51. Taylor, Rod S., Kate E. Ashton, Tiffany Moxham, Lee Hooper, and Shah Ebrahim. 2011. "Reduced Dietary Salt for the Prevention of Cardiovascular Disease: A Meta-Analysis of Randomized Controlled Trials (Cochrane Review)." *American Journal of Hypertension* 24 (8): 843–53.
52. O'Donnell, Martin J., Salim Yusuf, Andrew Mente, Peggy

Gao, Johannes F. Mann, Koon Teo, Matthew McQueen, et al. 2011. "Urinary Sodium and Potassium Excretion and Risk of Cardiovascular Events." *JAMA: The Journal of the American Medical Association* 306 (20): 2229–38.

53. Moyer, Melinda Wenner. 2011. "It's Time to End the War on Salt." Scientific American, July 8, 2011. https://www.scientificamerican.com/article/its-time-to-end-the-war-on-salt/.

54. Rousset, Bernard, Corinne Dupuy, Françoise Miot, and Jacques Dumont. 2015. "Chapter 2 Thyroid Hormone Synthesis And Secretion." In *Endotext*, edited by Kenneth R. Feingold, Bradley Anawalt, Alison Boyce, George Chrousos, Kathleen Dungan, Ashley Grossman, Jerome M. Hershman, et al. South Dartmouth (MA): MDText.com, Inc.

55. Xavier, A. R., M. A. R. Garófalo, R. H. Migliorini, and I. C. Kettelhut. 2003. "Dietary Sodium Restriction Exacerbates Age-Related Changes in Rat Adipose Tissue and Liver Lipogenesis." *Metabolism: Clinical and Experimental* 52 (8): 1072–77.

56. Horton, R., N. J. Rothwell, and M. J. Stock. 1988. "Chronic Inhibition of GABA Transaminase Results in Activation of Thermogenesis and Brown Fat in the Rat." *General Pharmacology* 19 (3): 403–5.

57. Dewasmes, G., N. Loos, S. Delanaud, D. Dewasmes, and A. Géloën. 2003. "Activation of Brown Adipose Tissue Thermogenesis Increases Slow Wave Sleep in Rat." *Neuroscience Letters* 339 (3): 207–10.

58. Wang, Gordon, Brian Grone, Damien Colas, Lior Appelbaum, and Philippe Mourrain. 2011. "Synaptic Plasticity

in Sleep: Learning, Homeostasis and Disease." *Trends in Neurosciences* 34 (9): 452–63.

59. Godek, Sandra Fowkes, Chris Peduzzi, Richard Burkholder, Steve Condon, Gary Dorshimer, and Arthur R. Bartolozzi. 2010. "Sweat Rates, Sweat Sodium Concentrations, and Sodium Losses in 3 Groups of Professional Football Players." *Journal of Athletic Training* 45 (4): 364–71.
60. *The Salt Fix by Dr. James DiNicolantonio: 9780451496966 | PenguinRandomHouse.com: Books.*

Chapter 3 - Sugar

1. Brown, William Redman, Arild Edsten Hansen, George Oswald Burr, and Irvine McQuarrie. 1938. "Effects of Prolonged Use of Extremely Low-Fat Diet on an Adult Human Subject." *The Journal of Nutrition* 16 (6): 511–24.
2. Bacon, Francis. 1898. *The Advancement of Learning.* Macmillan & Company, Limited.
3. Burton, Robert. 2008. *On Being Certain: Believing You Are Right Even When You're Not.* 1st ed. St. Martin's Press.
4. *Scientific American*. 2008. "The Certainty Bias: A Potentially Dangerous Mental Flaw," October 9, 2008. https://www.scientificamerican.com/article/the-certainty-bias/.
5. "William James." 2014. August 18, 2014. https://www.giffordlectures.org/lecturers/william-james.
6. Smith, William, and Rajendrani Mukhopadhyay. 2012. "Essential Fatty Acids: The Work of George and Mildred

Burr." *The Journal of Biological Chemistry* 287 (42): 35439–41.

7. Bernays, Edward, and Mark Crispin Miller. 2004. *Propaganda*. Ig Publishing.

8. "Obesity and Overweight." n.d. Accessed November 13, 2020. https://www.who.int/news-room/fact-sheets/detail/obesity-and-overweight.

9. Ravnskov, Uffe, Michel de Lorgeril, David M. Diamond, Rokuro Hama, Tomohito Hamazaki, Björn Hammarskjöld, Niamh Hynes, et al. 2018. "LDL-C Does Not Cause Cardiovascular Disease: A Comprehensive Review of the Current Literature." *Expert Review of Clinical Pharmacology* 11 (10): 959–70.

10. Barclay, Alan W., and Jennie Brand-Miller. 2011. "The Australian Paradox: A Substantial Decline in Sugars Intake over the Same Timeframe That Overweight and Obesity Have Increased." *Nutrients* 3 (4): 491–504.

11. Berg, Jeremy M., John L. Tymoczko, and Lubert Stryer. 2002. *Each Organ Has a Unique Metabolic Profile*. W H Freeman.

12. Golay, A., A. F. Allaz, Y. Morel, N. de Tonnac, S. Tankova, and G. Reaven. 1996. "Similar Weight Loss with Low- or High-Carbohydrate Diets." *The American Journal of Clinical Nutrition* 63 (2): 174–78.

13. Libretexts. 2016. "5.2: Carbohydrate Structures." Libretexts. August 5, 2016. https://chem.libretexts.org/Courses/University_of_Kentucky/UK%3A_CHE_103_-_Chemistry_for_Allied_Health_(Soult)/Chapters/Chapter_5%3A_Properties_of_Compounds/5.2%3A_Carbohydrate_Structures.

14. "Carbohydrates." n.d. Accessed March 31, 2021. https://dlc.dcccd.edu/biology1-3/carbohydrates.
15. Libretexts. 2017. "4.4: Nucleic Acids." Libretexts. March 26, 2017. https://bio.libretexts.org/Courses/University_of_California_Davis/BIS_2A%3A_Introductory_Biology_(Easlon)/Readings/04.4%3A_Nucleic_Acids.
16. "Carbohydrates." n.d. Accessed March 31, 2021. http://chemed.chem.purdue.edu/genchem/topicreview/bp/1biochem/carbo5.html.
17. "Gluconeogenesis." n.d. Accessed March 31, 2021. https://www.sciencedirect.com/topics/biochemistry-genetics-and-molecular-biology/gluconeogenesis.
18. Stone, Matt. 2010. "The Catecholamine Honeymoon - 180 Degree Health." June 10, 2010. https://180degreehealth.com/the-catecholamine-honeymoon/.
19. Ahmadi-Abhari, Sara, Robert N. Luben, Natasha Powell, Amit Bhaniani, Rajiv Chowdhury, Nicholas J. Wareham, Nita G. Forouhi, and Kay-Tee Khaw. 2014. "Dietary Intake of Carbohydrates and Risk of Type 2 Diabetes: The European Prospective Investigation into Cancer-Norfolk Study." *The British Journal of Nutrition* 111 (2): 342–52.
20. Brundin, T., and J. Wahren. 1993. "Whole Body and Splanchnic Oxygen Consumption and Blood Flow after Oral Ingestion of Fructose or Glucose." *The American Journal of Physiology* 264 (4 Pt 1): E504–13.
21. Cozma, Adrian I., John L. Sievenpiper, Russell J. de Souza, Laura Chiavaroli, Vanessa Ha, D. David Wang, Arash Mirrahimi, et al. 2012. "Effect of Fructose on Glycemic Control in Diabetes: A Systematic Review and Meta-Analysis

of Controlled Feeding Trials." *Diabetes Care* 35 (7): 1611–20.

22. DeCasien, Alex R., Scott A. Williams, and James P. Higham. 2017. "Primate Brain Size Is Predicted by Diet but Not Sociality." *Nature Ecology & Evolution* 1 (5): 112.

23. Wikipedia contributors. 2021. "Frugivore." Wikipedia, The Free Encyclopedia. March 18, 2021. https://en.wikipedia.org/w/index.php?title=Frugivore&oldid=1012820799.

24. Team FPS. n.d. "Ray Peat, PhD on Thyroid, Temperature, Pulse, and TSH." Accessed March 31, 2021. https://www.functionalps.com/blog/2012/03/25/ray-peat-phd-on-thyroid-temperature-pulse-and-tsh/comment-page-1/.

25. Kuoppala, Ali. n.d. "Thyroid Boosters: 6 Supplements to Increase T3 & T4." Accessed March 31, 2021. https://anabolicmen.com/thyroid-supplements/.

26. "Fructose as a Dieting Tool: 100g Fructose Per Day Exert Sign. Protein Sparing Effects & Ameliorate the Decline in Thyroid Hormones During Starvation Diet in the Obese." n.d. Accessed March 31, 2021. https://suppversity.blogspot.com/2014/10/fructose-as-dieting-tool-100g-fructose.html.

27. Hendler, R., and A. A. Bonde. 1990. "Effects of Sucrose on Resting Metabolic Rate, Nitrogen Balance, Leucine Turnover and Oxidation during Weight Loss with Low Calorie Diets." *International Journal of Obesity* 14 (11): 927–38.

28. Gelfand, Robert A., and Robert S. Sherwin. "Nitrogen conservation in starvation revisited: Protein sparing with intravenous fructose." Metabolism 35.1 (1986): 37-44.

29. Siyuan Xia, Ruiting Lin, Lingtao Jin, Liang Zhao, Hee-Bum Kang, Yaozhu Pan, Shuangping Liu, Guoqing Qian, Zhiyu Qian, Evmorfia Konstantakou, Baotong Zhang, Jin-

Tang Dong, Young Rock Chung, Omar Abdel-Wahab, Taha Merghoub, Lu Zhou, Ragini R. Kudchadkar, David H. Lawson, Hanna J. Khoury, Fadlo R. Khuri, Lawrence H. Boise, Sagar Lonial, Benjamin H. Lee, Brian P. Pollack, Jack L. Arbiser, Jun Fan, Qun-Ying Lei, Jing Chen. **Prevention of Dietary-Fat-Fueled Ketogenesis Attenuates BRAF V600E Tumor Growth.** *Cell Metabolism*, 2017; DOI: 10.1016/j.cmet.2016.12.010

30. Pierotti, Marco A., Gabriella Sozzi, and Carlo M. Croce. 2003. *Mechanisms of Oncogene Activation*. BC Decker.
31. Science X staff. 2010. "Researchers Find Leukemia Cells Metabolize Fat to Avoid Cell Death." Medical Xpress. January 27, 2010. https://medicalxpress.com/news/2010-01-leukemia-cells-metabolize-fat-cell.html.
32. Currie, Erin, Almut Schulze, Rudolf Zechner, Tobias C. Walther, and Robert V. Farese Jr. 2013. "Cellular Fatty Acid Metabolism and Cancer." *Cell Metabolism* 18 (2): 153–61.
33. Choi, Yeon-Kyung, and Keun-Gyu Park. 2018. "Targeting Glutamine Metabolism for Cancer Treatment." *Biomolecules & Therapeutics* 26 (1): 19–28.
34. "Nonalcoholic Fatty Liver Disease (NAFLD)." 2017. July 31, 2017. https://liverfoundation.org/for-patients/about-the-liver/diseases-of-the-liver/non-alcoholic-fatty-liver-disease/.
35. Anundi, I., J. King, D. A. Owen, H. Schneider, J. J. Lemasters, and R. G. Thurman. 1987. "Fructose Prevents Hypoxic Cell Death in Liver." *The American Journal of Physiology* 253 (3 Pt 1): G390–96.
36. Kuoppala, Ali. n.d. "Choline and Testosterone: Why Deficiency Hurts Hormones." Accessed March 31, 2021.

https://anabolicmen.com/choline-deficiency/.

37. Best, C. H., and W. S. Hartroft. 1949. "Liver Damage Produced by Feeding Alcohol or Sugar and Its Prevention by Choline." *British Medical Journal* 2 (4635): 1002–6, pl.

38. Pan, Meihui, Arthur I. Cederbaum, Yuan-Li Zhang, Henry N. Ginsberg, Kevin Jon Williams, and Edward A. Fisher. 2004. "Lipid Peroxidation and Oxidant Stress Regulate Hepatic Apolipoprotein B Degradation and VLDL Production." *The Journal of Clinical Investigation* 113 (9): 1277–87.

39. Corbin, Karen D., and Steven H. Zeisel. 2012. "Choline Metabolism Provides Novel Insights into Nonalcoholic Fatty Liver Disease and Its Progression." *Current Opinion in Gastroenterology* 28 (2): 159–65.

40. Wallace, Taylor C., Michael McBurney, and Victor L. Fulgoni 3rd. 2014. "Multivitamin/mineral Supplement Contribution to Micronutrient Intakes in the United States, 2007-2010." *Journal of the American College of Nutrition* 33 (2): 94–102.

41. "Liver Disease Statistics." 2017. October 26, 2017. https://liverfoundation.org/liver-disease-statistics/.

42. Harvey, Cliff J. D. C., Grant M. Schofield, and Micalla Williden. 2018. "The Use of Nutritional Supplements to Induce Ketosis and Reduce Symptoms Associated with Keto-Induction: A Narrative Review." *PeerJ* 6 (March): e4488.

43. Chidakel, A., D. Mentuccia, and F. S. Celi. 2005. "Peripheral Metabolism of Thyroid Hormone and Glucose Homeostasis." *Thyroid: Official Journal of the American Thyroid Association* 15 (8): 899–903.

44. Cahoreau, Claire, Danièle Klett, and Yves Combarnous.

2015. "Structure-Function Relationships of Glycoprotein Hormones and Their Subunits' Ancestors." *Frontiers in Endocrinology* 6 (February): 26.

45. Spaulding, S. W., I. J. Chopra, R. S. Sherwin, and S. S. Lyall. 1976. "Effect of Caloric Restriction and Dietary Composition of Serum T3 and Reverse T3 in Man." *The Journal of Clinical Endocrinology and Metabolism* 42 (1): 197–200.

46. McCarty, M. F. 1995. "Central Insulin May up-Regulate Thyroid Activity by Suppressing Neuropeptide Y Release in the Paraventricular Nucleus." *Medical Hypotheses* 45 (2): 193–99.

47. Wheless, James W. 2008. "History of the Ketogenic Diet." *Epilepsia* 49 Suppl 8 (November): 3–5.

48. Bisschop, P. H., H. P. Sauerwein, E. Endert, and J. A. Romijn. 2001. "Isocaloric Carbohydrate Deprivation Induces Protein Catabolism despite a Low T3-Syndrome in Healthy Men." *Clinical Endocrinology* 54 (1): 75–80.

49. Azizi, F. 1978. "Effect of Dietary Composition on Fasting-Induced Changes in Serum Thyroid Hormones and Thyrotropin." *Metabolism: Clinical and Experimental* 27 (8): 935–42.

50. Burman, K. D., R. C. Dimond, G. S. Harvey, J. T. O'Brian, L. P. Georges, J. Bruton, F. D. Wright, and L. Wartofsky. 1979. "Glucose Modulation of Alterations in Serum Iodothyronine Concentrations Induced by Fasting." *Metabolism: Clinical and Experimental* 28 (4): 291–99.

51. Burke, Louise M., Bente Kiens, and John L. Ivy. 2004. "Carbohydrates and Fat for Training and Recovery." *Journal of Sports Sciences* 22 (1): 15–30.

52. Langfort, J., R. Zarzeczny, W. Pilis, K. Nazar, and H. Kaciuba-Uścitko. 1997. "The Effect of a Low-Carbohydrate Diet on Performance, Hormonal and Metabolic Responses to a 30-S Bout of Supramaximal Exercise." *European Journal of Applied Physiology and Occupational Physiology* 76 (2): 128–33.
53. Maughan, R. J., P. L. Greenhaff, J. B. Leiper, D. Ball, C. P. Lambert, and M. Gleeson. 1997. "Diet Composition and the Performance of High-Intensity Exercise." *Journal of Sports Sciences* 15 (3): 265–75.
54. Pinckaers, Philippe J. M., Tyler A. Churchward-Venne, David Bailey, and Luc J. C. van Loon. 2017. "Ketone Bodies and Exercise Performance: The Next Magic Bullet or Merely Hype?" *Sports Medicine* 47 (3): 383–91.
55. Cox, Pete J., Tom Kirk, Tom Ashmore, Kristof Willerton, Rhys Evans, Alan Smith, Andrew J. Murray, et al. 2016. "Nutritional Ketosis Alters Fuel Preference and Thereby Endurance Performance in Athletes." *Cell Metabolism* 24 (2): 256–68.
56. Zinn, Caryn, Matthew Wood, Mikki Williden, Simon Chatterton, and Ed Maunder. 2017. "Ketogenic Diet Benefits Body Composition and Well-Being but Not Performance in a Pilot Case Study of New Zealand Endurance Athletes." *Journal of the International Society of Sports Nutrition* 14 (July): 22.
57. Urbain, Paul, Lena Strom, Lena Morawski, Anja Wehrle, Peter Deibert, and Hartmut Bertz. 2017. "Impact of a 6-Week Non-Energy-Restricted Ketogenic Diet on Physical Fitness, Body Composition and Biochemical Parameters in Healthy Adults." *Nutrition & Metabolism* 14 (February): 17.
58. Burke, Louise M., Megan L. Ross, Laura A. Garvican-

Lewis, Marijke Welvaert, Ida A. Heikura, Sara G. Forbes, Joanne G. Mirtschin, et al. 2017. "Low Carbohydrate, High Fat Diet Impairs Exercise Economy and Negates the Performance Benefit from Intensified Training in Elite Race Walkers." *The Journal of Physiology* 595 (9): 2785–2807.

59. Phinney, Stephen D. 2004. "Ketogenic Diets and Physical Performance." *Nutrition & Metabolism* 1 (1): 2.
60. "High-Fat Diet Affects Physical and Memory Abilities." 2009. August 13, 2009. https://www.cam.ac.uk/research/news/high-fat-diet-affects-physical-and-memory-abilities.
61. Tagliabue, Anna, Simona Bertoli, Claudia Trentani, Paola Borrelli, and Pierangelo Veggiotti. 2012. "Effects of the Ketogenic Diet on Nutritional Status, Resting Energy Expenditure, and Substrate Oxidation in Patients with Medically Refractory Epilepsy: A 6-Month Prospective Observational Study." *Clinical Nutrition* 31 (2): 246–49.
62. Harber, Matthew P., Simon Schenk, Ariel L. Barkan, and Jeffrey F. Horowitz. 2005. "Effects of Dietary Carbohydrate Restriction with High Protein Intake on Protein Metabolism and the Somatotropic Axis." *The Journal of Clinical Endocrinology and Metabolism* 90 (9): 5175–81.
63. Bravata, Dena M., Lisa Sanders, Jane Huang, Harlan M. Krumholz, Ingram Olkin, Christopher D. Gardner, and Dawn M. Bravata. 2003. "Efficacy and Safety of Low-Carbohydrate Diets: A Systematic Review." *JAMA: The Journal of the American Medical Association* 289 (14): 1837–50.
64. Boden, Guenther, Karin Sargrad, Carol Homko, Maria Mozzoli, and T. Peter Stein. 2005. "Effect of a Low-

Carbohydrate Diet on Appetite, Blood Glucose Levels, and Insulin Resistance in Obese Patients with Type 2 Diabetes." *Annals of Internal Medicine* 142 (6): 403–11.

65. Astrup, Arne, Arne Astrup, Benjamin Buemann, Anne Flint, and Anne Raben. 2002. "Low-Fat Diets and Energy Balance: How Does the Evidence Stand in 2002?" *The Proceedings of the Nutrition Society* 61 (2): 299–309.

66. Yang, M. U., and T. B. Van Itallie. 1976. "Composition of Weight Lost during Short-Term Weight Reduction. Metabolic Responses of Obese Subjects to Starvation and Low-Calorie Ketogenic and Nonketogenic Diets." *The Journal of Clinical Investigation* 58 (3): 722–30.

67. Murphy, E. Angela, Kandy T. Velazquez, and Kyle M. Herbert. 2015. "Influence of High-Fat Diet on Gut Microbiota: A Driving Force for Chronic Disease Risk." *Current Opinion in Clinical Nutrition and Metabolic Care* 18 (5): 515–20.

68. Zhang, Mei, and Xiao-Jiao Yang. 2016. "Effects of a High Fat Diet on Intestinal Microbiota and Gastrointestinal Diseases." *World Journal of Gastroenterology: WJG* 22 (40): 8905–9.

69. Brown, G. K. 2000. "Glucose Transporters: Structure, Function and Consequences of Deficiency." *Journal of Inherited Metabolic Disease* 23 (3): 237–46.

70. Phinney, S. D., B. R. Bistrian, R. R. Wolfe, and G. L. Blackburn. 1983. "The Human Metabolic Response to Chronic Ketosis without Caloric Restriction: Physical and Biochemical Adaptation." *Metabolism: Clinical and Experimental* 32 (8): 757–68.

71. Harber, Matthew P., Simon Schenk, Ariel L. Barkan, and Jeffrey F. Horowitz. 2005. "Alterations in Carbohydrate Metabolism in Response to Short-Term Dietary Carbohydrate Restriction." *American Journal of Physiology. Endocrinology and Metabolism* 289 (2): E306–12.

72. Sandu, Oana, Keying Song, Weijing Cai, Feng Zheng, Jaime Uribarri, and Helen Vlassara. 2005. "Insulin Resistance and Type 2 Diabetes in High-Fat-Fed Mice Are Linked to High Glycotoxin Intake." *Diabetes* 54 (8): 2314–19.

73. Kusunoki, M., G. J. Cooney, T. Hara, and L. H. Storlien. 1995. "Amelioration of High-Fat Feeding-Induced Insulin Resistance in Skeletal Muscle with the Antiglucocorticoid RU486." *Diabetes* 44 (6): 718–20.

74. Ikemoto, S., Kimberly S. THOMPSONt, Mayumi Takahashi, H. Itakura, M. DANIEL LANEt, and O. Ezaki. 2005. "High Fat Diet-Induced Hyperglycemia : Prevention by Low Level Expression of a Glucose Transporter (GLUT 4) Minigene in Transgenic Mice (Insulin Resistance / Type 2 Diabetes)." https://www.semanticscholar.org/paper/7066b17637d4e5e007f521cd42d1fe8e6393f54a.

75. Felber, J. P., E. Ferrannini, A. Golay, H. U. Meyer, D. Theibaud, B. Curchod, E. Maeder, E. Jequier, and R. A. DeFronzo. 1987. "Role of Lipid Oxidation in Pathogenesis of Insulin Resistance of Obesity and Type II Diabetes." *Diabetes* 36 (11): 1341–50.

76. n.d. http://europepmc.org/article/med/7621976.

77. Dobbins, Robert L., Lidia S. Szczepaniak, Jeff Myhill, Yoshifumi Tamura, Hiroshi Uchino, Adria Giacca, and J. Denis McGarry. 2002. "The Composition of Dietary Fat

Directly Influences Glucose-Stimulated Insulin Secretion in Rats." *Diabetes* 51 (6): 1825–33.

78. Bantle, J. P., J. E. Swanson, W. Thomas, and D. C. Laine. 1993. "Metabolic Effects of Dietary Sucrose in Type II Diabetic Subjects." *Diabetes Care* 16 (9): 1301–5.

79. Mithal, A., J-P Bonjour, S. Boonen, P. Burckhardt, H. Degens, G. El Hajj Fuleihan, R. Josse, et al. 2013. "Impact of Nutrition on Muscle Mass, Strength, and Performance in Older Adults." *Osteoporosis International: A Journal Established as Result of Cooperation between the European Foundation for Osteoporosis and the National Osteoporosis Foundation of the USA* 24 (5): 1555–66.

80. Hahn, T. J., L. R. Halstead, and D. C. DeVivo. 1979. "Disordered Mineral Metabolism Produced by Ketogenic Diet Therapy." *Calcified Tissue International* 28 (1): 17–22.

81. Hahn, T. J., L. R. Halstead, and D. C. DeVivo. 1979. "Disordered Mineral Metabolism Produced by Ketogenic Diet Therapy." *Calcified Tissue International* 28 (1): 17–22.

82. Bergqvist, A. G. Christina, Claire M. Chee, Lisa Lutchka, Jack Rychik, and Virginia A. Stallings. 2003. "Selenium Deficiency Associated with Cardiomyopathy: A Complication of the Ketogenic Diet." *Epilepsia* 44 (4): 618–20.

83. Fery, F., P. Bourdoux, J. Christophe, and E. O. Balasse. 1982. "Hormonal and Metabolic Changes Induced by an Isocaloric Isoproteinic Ketogenic Diet in Healthy Subjects." *Diabete & Metabolisme* 8 (4): 299–305.

84. Hamburg, Naomi M., Craig J. McMackin, Alex L. Huang, Sherene M. Shenouda, Michael E. Widlansky, Eberhard Schulz, Noyan Gokce, Neil B. Ruderman, John F. Keaney Jr,

and Joseph A. Vita. 2007. "Physical Inactivity Rapidly Induces Insulin Resistance and Microvascular Dysfunction in Healthy Volunteers." *Arteriosclerosis, Thrombosis, and Vascular Biology* 27 (12): 2650–56.

85. https://www.ncbi.nlm.nih.gov/pmc/articles/PMC2713647/

86. https://journals.physiology.org/doi/full/10.1152/ajpendo.00590.2009

Chapter 4 - PUFA

1. Mercola, Joseph. 2017. Fat for Fuel: *A Revolutionary Diet to Combat Cancer, Boost Brain Power, and Increase Your Energy*. Hay House, Inc.

2. Ramsey, Drew, and Tyler Graham. 2012. "How Vegetable Oils Replaced Animal Fats in the American Diet." *The Atlantic*, April 26, 2012. https://www.theatlantic.com/health/archive/2012/04/how-vegetable-oils-replaced-animal-fats-in-the-american-diet/256155/.

3. "Facts about Polyunsaturated Fats." n.d. Accessed March 31, 2021. https://medlineplus.gov/ency/patientinstructions/000747.htm.

4. "Good Fats vs. Bad Fats: Get the Skinny on Fat." n.d. Accessed March 31, 2021. https://www.webmd.com/diet/obesity/features/skinny-fat-good-fats-bad-fats.

5. "Healthy for Good." n.d. Accessed March 31, 2021. https://www.heart.org/en/healthy-living.

6. Roussell, Mike. 2014. "Ask the Diet Doctor: Importance of Polyunsaturated Fat." Shape. December 9, 2014. https://

www.shape.com/healthy-eating/diet-tips/ask-diet-doctor-importance-polyunsaturated-fat.

7. "Ask the Expert: Healthy Fats." 2012. June 21, 2012. https://www.hsph.harvard.edu/nutritionsource/2012/06/21/ask-the-expert-healthy-fats/.
8. "Fats: The Good, the Bad & the Ugly." n.d. Accessed March 31, 2021. https://www.unitypoint.org/livewell/article.aspx?id=a08a02ac-918c-493d-ba8a-6722940599d6.
9. "Fats." n.d. Accessed March 31, 2021. https://www.diabetes.org/healthy-living/recipes-nutrition/eating-well/fats.
10. Yin, Huiyong, Joshua D. Brooks, Ling Gao, Ned A. Porter, and Jason D. Morrow. 2007. "Identification of Novel Autoxidation Products of the Omega-3 Fatty Acid Eicosapentaenoic Acid in Vitro and in Vivo." *The Journal of Biological Chemistry* 282 (41): 29890–901.
11. Davis, Todd A., Ling Gao, Huiyong Yin, Jason D. Morrow, and Ned A. Porter. 2006. "In Vivo and in Vitro Lipid Peroxidation of Arachidonate Esters: The Effect of Fish Oil Omega-3 Lipids on Product Distribution." *Journal of the American Chemical Society* 128 (46): 14897–904.
12. Lefkowith, J. B., A. Morrison, V. Lee, and M. Rogers. 1990. "Manipulation of the Acute Inflammatory Response by Dietary Polyunsaturated Fatty Acid Modulation." *Journal of Immunology* 145 (5): 1523–29.
13. http://europepmc.org/article/MED/2188748
14. Wright, J. R., Jr, J. B. Lefkowith, G. Schreiner, and P. E. Lacy. 1988. "Essential Fatty Acid Deficiency Prevents Multiple Low-Dose Streptozotocin-Induced Diabetes in CD-1

Mice." *Proceedings of the National Academy of Sciences of the United States of America* 85 (16): 6137–41.

15. Wright, J. R., Jr, B. Haliburton, H. Russell, M. Henry, R. Fraser, and H. W. Cook. 1991. "The Anti-Diabetogenic Effect of Essential Fatty Acid Deficiency in Multiple Low-Dose Streptozotocin-Treated Mice Persists If Essential Fatty Acid Repletion Occurs outside of a Brief Window of Susceptibility." *Diabetologia* 34 (10): 709–14.
16. Wright, J. R., Jr, B. Haliburton, H. Russell, M. Henry, R. Fraser, and H. W. Cook. 1991. "The Anti-Diabetogenic Effect of Essential Fatty Acid Deficiency in Multiple Low-Dose Streptozotocin-Treated Mice Persists If Essential Fatty Acid Repletion Occurs outside of a Brief Window of Susceptibility." *Diabetologia* 34 (10): 709–14.
17. Pamplona, R., M. Portero-Otín, C. Ruiz, R. Gredilla, A. Herrero, and G. Barja. 2000. "Double Bond Content of Phospholipids and Lipid Peroxidation Negatively Correlate with Maximum Longevity in the Heart of Mammals." *Mechanisms of Ageing and Development* 112 (3): 169–83.
18. https://courses.washington.edu/conj/bess/cholesterol/liver.html
19. McDermott, Annette. 2017. "HDL vs. LDL Cholesterol: What's the Difference?" January 23, 2017. https://www.healthline.com/health/hdl-vs-ldl-cholesterol#hdl-vs-ldl.
20. Benassayag, C., V. Rigourd, T. M. Mignot, J. Hassid, M. J. Leroy, B. Robert, C. Civel, et al. 1999. "Does High Polyunsaturated Free Fatty Acid Level at the Feto-Maternal Interface Alter Steroid Hormone Message during Pregnancy?" *Prostaglandins, Leukotrienes, and Essential Fatty*

Acids 60 (5-6): 393–99.

21. Valencak, Teresa G., and Thomas Ruf. 2007. "N-3 Polyunsaturated Fatty Acids Impair Lifespan but Have No Role for Metabolism." *Aging Cell* 6 (1): 15–25.
22. Speake, B. K., S. Cerolini, A. Maldjian, and R. C. Noble. 1997. "The Preferential Mobilisation of C20 and C22 Polyunsaturated Fatty Acids from the Adipose Tissue of the Chick Embryo: Potential Implications Regarding the Provision of Essential Fatty Acids for Neural Development." *Biochimica et Biophysica Acta* 1345 (3): 317–26.
23. Easton, A. S., and P. A. Fraser. 1998. "Arachidonic Acid Increases Cerebral Microvascular Permeability by Free Radicals in Single Pial Microvessels of the Anaesthetized Rat." *The Journal of Physiology* 507 (Pt 2) (March): 541–47.
24. Dhein, Stefan, Bjela Michaelis, and Friedrich-Wilhelm Mohr. 2005. "Antiarrhythmic and Electrophysiological Effects of Long-Chain Omega-3 Polyunsaturated Fatty Acids." *Naunyn-Schmiedeberg's Archives of Pharmacology* 371 (3): 202–11.
25. Volek, J. S., W. J. Kraemer, J. A. Bush, T. Incledon, and M. Boetes. 1997. "Testosterone and Cortisol in Relationship to Dietary Nutrients and Resistance Exercise." *Journal of Applied Physiology* 82 (1): 49–54.
26. http://europepmc.org/article/med/8960090
27. Calder, Philip C. 2010. "Omega-3 Fatty Acids and Inflammatory Processes." *Nutrients* 2 (3): 355–74.
28. Calder, Philip C. 2010. "Omega-3 Fatty Acids and Inflammatory Processes." *Nutrients* 2 (3): 355–74.
29. https://link.springer.com/article/10.1007/s003830100589

30. Wang, Yutong, and John F. Oram. 2002. "Unsaturated Fatty Acids Inhibit Cholesterol Efflux from Macrophages by Increasing Degradation of ATP-Binding Cassette Transporter A1 *." *The Journal of Biological Chemistry* 277 (7): 5692–97.

31. Simopoulos, A. P. 2002. "The Importance of the Ratio of Omega-6/omega-3 Essential Fatty Acids." *Biomedicine & Pharmacotherapy = Biomedecine & Pharmacotherapie* 56 (8): 365–79.

32. Bélanger, A., A. Locong, C. Noel, L. Cusan, A. Dupont, J. Prévost, S. Caron, and J. Sévigny. 1989. "Influence of Diet on Plasma Steroids and Sex Hormone-Binding Globulin Levels in Adult Men." *Journal of Steroid Biochemistry* 32 (6): 829–33.

33. Salvayre, Robert, Nathalie Auge, Herve Benoist, and Anne Negre-Salvayre. 2002. "Oxidized Low-Density Lipoprotein-Induced Apoptosis." *Biochimica et Biophysica Acta* 1585 (2–3): 213–21.

34. Eaves, P.H., Molaison, L.J., Black, C.L. et al. A comparison of five commercial solvents for extraction of cottonseed. *J Am Oil Chem Soc* 29, 88–94 (1952). https://doi.org/10.1007/BF02648783

35. Awada, Manar, Christophe O. Soulage, Anne Meynier, Cyrille Debard, Pascale Plaisancié, Bérengère Benoit, Grégory Picard, et al. 2012. "Dietary Oxidized N-3 PUFA Induce Oxidative Stress and Inflammation: Role of Intestinal Absorption of 4-HHE and Reactivity in Intestinal Cells." *Journal of Lipid Research* 53 (10): 2069–80.

36. Song, J. H., K. Fujimoto, and T. Miyazawa. 2000. "Polyunsaturated (n-3) Fatty Acids Susceptible to Peroxidation Are Increased in Plasma and Tissue Lipids

of Rats Fed Docosahexaenoic Acid-Containing Oils." The *Journal of Nutrition* 130 (12): 3028–33.

37. Sakamoto, N., T. Nishiike, H. Iguchi, and K. Sakamoto. 2000. "Effects of Eicosapentaenoic Acid Intake on Plasma Fibrinolytic and Coagulation Activity by Using Physical Load in the Young." *Nutrition* 16 (1): 11–14.

38. Pan, Meihui, Arthur I. Cederbaum, Yuan-Li Zhang, Henry N. Ginsberg, Kevin Jon Williams, and Edward A. Fisher. 2004. "Lipid Peroxidation and Oxidant Stress Regulate Hepatic Apolipoprotein B Degradation and VLDL Production." *The Journal of Clinical Investigation* 113 (9): 1277–87.

39. Okuyama, Harumi, Peter H. Langsjoen, Naoki Ohara, Yoko Hashimoto, Tomohito Hamazaki, Satoshi Yoshida, Tetsuyuki Kobayashi, and Alena M. Langsjoen. 2016. "Medicines and Vegetable Oils as Hidden Causes of Cardiovascular Disease and Diabetes." *Pharmacology* 98 (3-4): 134–70.

40. https://www.nature.com/articles/ajg201144

41. Cardoso, Cristina Ribeiro Barros, Maria Aparecida Souza, Eloísa Amália Vieira Ferro, Sílvio Favoreto Jr, and Janethe Deolina Oliviera Pena. 2004. "Influence of Topical Administration of N-3 and N-6 Essential and N-9 Nonessential Fatty Acids on the Healing of Cutaneous Wounds." *Wound Repair and Regeneration: Official Publication of the Wound Healing Society [and] the European Tissue Repair Society* 12 (2): 235–43.

42. Dirix, C. E. H., G. Hornstra, and J. G. Nijhuis. 2009. "Fetal Learning and Memory: Weak Associations with the Early Essential Polyunsaturated Fatty Acid Status." *Prostaglandins,*

Leukotrienes, and Essential Fatty Acids 80 (4): 207–12.

43. Zhang, Bin-Xian, Xiuye Ma, Wanke Zhang, Chih-Ko Yeh, Alan Lin, Jian Luo, Eugene A. Sprague, Russell H. Swerdlow, and Michael S. Katz. 2006. "Polyunsaturated Fatty Acids Mobilize Intracellular Ca2+ in NT2 Human Teratocarcinoma Cells by Causing Release of Ca2+ from Mitochondria." *American Journal of Physiology. Cell Physiology* 290 (5): C1321–33.
44. Bruder, Eric D., Dennis L. Ball, Theodore L. Goodfriend, and Hershel Raff. 2003. "An Oxidized Metabolite of Linoleic Acid Stimulates Corticosterone Production by Rat Adrenal Cells." *American Journal of Physiology. Regulatory, Integrative and Comparative Physiology* 284 (6): R1631–35.
45. Malhotra, Aseem, Rita F. Redberg, and Pascal Meier. 2017. "Saturated Fat Does Not Clog the Arteries: Coronary Heart Disease Is a Chronic Inflammatory Condition, the Risk of Which Can Be Effectively Reduced from Healthy Lifestyle Interventions." *British Journal of Sports Medicine* 51 (15): 1111–12.
46. Katoh, Kazuo, Mami Asari, Hiroko Ishiwata, Yasuyuki Sasaki, and Yoshiaki Obara. 2004. "Saturated Fatty Acids Suppress Adrenocorticotropic Hormone (ACTH) Release from Rat Anterior Pituitary Cells in Vitro." *Comparative Biochemistry and Physiology. Part A, Molecular & Integrative Physiology* 137 (2): 357–64.
47. Volek, J. S., W. J. Kraemer, J. A. Bush, T. Incledon, and M. Boetes. 1997. "Testosterone and Cortisol in Relationship to Dietary Nutrients and Resistance Exercise." *Journal of Applied Physiology* 82 (1): 49–54.

48. Segarra, A. B., M. Ramirez, I. Banegas, F. Alba, F. Vives, M. de Gasparo, E. Ortega, E. Ruiz, and I. Prieto. 2008. "Dietary Fat Influences Testosterone, Cholesterol, Aminopeptidase A, and Blood Pressure in Male Rats." *Hormone and Metabolic Research = Hormon- Und Stoffwechselforschung = Hormones et Metabolisme* 40 (4): 289–91.

49. Biello, David. 2010. "Genetically Modified Crop on the Loose and Evolving in U.S. Midwest." *Scientific American*, August 6, 2010. https://www.scientificamerican.com/article/genetically-modified-crop/.

50. "10 Reasons to Avoid GMOs." 2020. January 25, 2020. https://www.responsibletechnology.org/for-parents/parents-tool-kit/10-reasons-to-avoid-gmos/.

51. "CornOil.pdf." n.d. https://corn.org/wp-content/uploads/2009/12/CornOil.pdf.

52. "Soy Report and Scorecard." 2009. May 18, 2009. https://www.cornucopia.org/research/soy-report-and-scorecard/.

53. Eaves, P. H., L. J. Molaison, C. L. Black, A. J. Crovetto, and E. L. D'Aquin. 1952. "A Comparison of Five Commercial Solvents for Extraction of Cottonseed." *Journal of the American Oil Chemists' Society* 29 (3): 88–94.

54. "Sodium Carbonate." n.d. Accessed March 31, 2021. https://www.encyclopedia.com/science-and-technology/chemistry/compounds-and-elements/sodium-carbonate.

55. Valencak, Teresa G., and Thomas Ruf. 2007. "N-3 Polyunsaturated Fatty Acids Impair Lifespan but Have No Role for Metabolism." *Aging Cell* 6 (1): 15–25.

56. Pamplona, R., M. Portero-Otín, C. Ruiz, R. Gredilla, A. Herrero, and G. Barja. 2000. "Double Bond Content of

Phospholipids and Lipid Peroxidation Negatively Correlate with Maximum Longevity in the Heart of Mammals." *Mechanisms of Ageing and Development* 112 (3): 169–83.

57. Okuyama, Harumi, Peter H. Langsjoen, Naoki Ohara, Yoko Hashimoto, Tomohito Hamazaki, Satoshi Yoshida, Tetsuyuki Kobayashi, and Alena M. Langsjoen. 2016. "Medicines and Vegetable Oils as Hidden Causes of Cardiovascular Disease and Diabetes." *Pharmacology* 98 (3-4): 134–70.
58. "Etomoxir." n.d. Accessed March 31, 2021. https://www.sciencedirect.com/topics/medicine-and-dentistry/etomoxir.
59. Steerenberg, P. A., P. K. Beekhof, E. J. M. Feskens, C. J. M. Lips, J. W. M. Höppener, and R. B. Beems. 2002. "Long-Term Effect of Fish Oil Diet on Basal and Stimulated Plasma Glucose and Insulin Levels in Ob/ob Mice." *Diabetes, Nutrition & Metabolism* 15 (4): 205–14.
60. Ramsden, Christopher E., Daisy Zamora, Boonseng Leelarthaepin, Sharon F. Majchrzak-Hong, Keturah R. Faurot, Chirayath M. Suchindran, Amit Ringel, John M. Davis, and Joseph R. Hibbeln. 2013. "Use of Dietary Linoleic Acid for Secondary Prevention of Coronary Heart Disease and Death: Evaluation of Recovered Data from the Sydney Diet Heart Study and Updated Meta-Analysis." *BMJ* 346 (February): e8707.
61. Volek, J. S., W. J. Kraemer, J. A. Bush, T. Incledon, and M. Boetes. 1997. "Testosterone and Cortisol in Relationship to Dietary Nutrients and Resistance Exercise." *Journal of Applied Physiology* 82 (1): 49–54.
62. Benassayag, C., V. Rigourd, T. M. Mignot, J. Hassid,

M. J. Leroy, B. Robert, C. Civel, et al. 1999. "Does High Polyunsaturated Free Fatty Acid Level at the Feto-Maternal Interface Alter Steroid Hormone Message during Pregnancy?" *Prostaglandins, Leukotrienes, and Essential Fatty Acids* 60 (5-6): 393–99.

63. http://europepmc.org/article/med/8960090

64. Bélanger, A., A. Locong, C. Noel, L. Cusan, A. Dupont, J. Prévost, S. Caron, and J. Sévigny. 1989. "Influence of Diet on Plasma Steroids and Sex Hormone-Binding Globulin Levels in Adult Men." *Journal of Steroid Biochemistry* 32 (6): 829–33.

65. Christeff, N., C. Michon, G. Goertz, J. Hassid, S. Matheron, P. M. Girard, J. P. Coulaud, and E. A. Nunez. 1988. "Abnormal Free Fatty Acids and Cortisol Concentrations in the Serum of AIDS Patients." *European Journal of Cancer & Clinical Oncology* 24 (7): 1179–83.

66. Altınterim, Başar. 2012. "ANTI-THYROID EFFECTS OF PUFAS (POLYUNSATURATED FATS) AND HERBS." *Trakya University Journal of Natural Sciences* 13 (2). http://dx.doi.org/.

67. Danforth, E., Jr, and A. Burger. 1984. "The Role of Thyroid Hormones in the Control of Energy Expenditure." *Clinics in Endocrinology and Metabolism* 13 (3): 581–95.

68. Clarke, S. D., and J. Hembree. 1990. "Inhibition of Triiodothyronine's Induction of Rat Liver Lipogenic Enzymes by Dietary Fat." *The Journal of Nutrition* 120 (6): 625–30.

Chapter 5 - Protein

1. "Proteins." 2015. May 10, 2015. https://basicbiology.net/

micro/biochemistry/protein.

2. Libretexts. 2018. "3.3A: Types and Functions of Proteins." Libretexts. July 5, 2018. https://bio.libretexts.org/Bookshelves/Introductory_and_General_Biology/Book%3A_General_Biology_(Boundless)/3%3A_Biological_Macromolecules/3.3%3A_Proteins/3.3A%3A_Types_and_Functions_of_Proteins.
3. DrJones. 2013. "GLYCINE." May 7, 2013. https://aminoacidstudies.org/glycine/.
4. Gusev, E. I., V. I. Skvortsova, S. A. Dambinova, K. S. Raevskiy, A. A. Alekseev, V. G. Bashkatova, A. V. Kovalenko, V. S. Kudrin, and E. V. Yakovleva. 2000. "Neuroprotective Effects of Glycine for Therapy of Acute Ischaemic Stroke." *Cerebrovascular Diseases* 10 (1): 49–60.
5. Díaz-Flores, Margarita, Miguel Cruz, Genoveva Duran-Reyes, Catarina Munguia-Miranda, Hilda Loza-Rodríguez, Evelyn Pulido-Casas, Nayeli Torres-Ramírez, et al. 2013. "Oral Supplementation with Glycine Reduces Oxidative Stress in Patients with Metabolic Syndrome, Improving Their Systolic Blood Pressure." *Canadian Journal of Physiology and Pharmacology* 91 (10): 855–60.
6. Yamadera, Wataru, Kentaro Inagawa, Shintaro Chiba, Makoto Bannai, Michio Takahashi, and Kazuhiko Nakayama. 2007. "Glycine Ingestion Improves Subjective Sleep Quality in Human Volunteers, Correlating with Polysomnographic Changes: Effects of Glycine on Polysomnography." *Sleep and Biological Rhythms* 5 (2): 126–31.
7. Bannai, Makoto, Nobuhiro Kawai, Kaori Ono, Keiko Nakahara, and Noboru Murakami. 2012. "The Effects of

Glycine on Subjective Daytime Performance in Partially Sleep-Restricted Healthy Volunteers." *Frontiers in Neurology* 3 (April): 61.

8. Arwert, L. I., J. B. Deijen, and M. L. Drent. 2003. "Effects of an Oral Mixture Containing Glycine, Glutamine and Niacin on Memory, GH and IGF-I Secretion in Middle-Aged and Elderly Subjects." *Nutritional Neuroscience* 6 (5): 269–75.
9. Kasai, K., M. Kobayashi, and S. I. Shimoda. 1978. "Stimulatory Effect of Glycine on Human Growth Hormone Secretion." *Metabolism: Clinical and Experimental* 27 (2): 201–8.
10. Kasai, K., H. Suzuki, T. Nakamura, H. Shiina, and S. I. Shimoda. 1980. "Glycine Stimulated Growth Hormone Release in Man." *Acta Endocrinologica* 93 (3): 283–86.
11. Petzke, K. J., K. L. Pisarchuk, Grigorov YuG, and V. Albrecht. 1987. "[The effect of oral administration of glycine on metabolism]." *Die Nahrung* 31 (3): 207–15.
12. Barakat, H. A., and A. H. Hamza. 2012. "Glycine Alleviates Liver Injury Induced by Deficiency in Methionine and or Choline in Rats." *European Review for Medical and Pharmacological Sciences* 16 (6): 728–36.
13. Senthilkumar, Rajagopal, Periyasamy Viswanathan, and Namasivayam Nalini. 2003. "Glycine Modulates Hepatic Lipid Accumulation in Alcohol-Induced Liver Injury." *Polish Journal of Pharmacology* 55 (4): 603–11.
14. Jones, Dr. 2016. "PROLINE." May 1, 2016. https://aminoacidstudies.org/l-proline/.
15. Kang, Ping, Lili Zhang, Yongqing Hou, Binying Ding, Dan Yi, Lei Wang, Huiling Zhu, Yulan Liu, Yulong Yin, and Guoyao

Wu. 2014. "Effects of L-Proline on the Growth Performance, and Blood Parameters in Weaned Lipopolysaccharide (LPS)-Challenged Pigs." *Asian-Australasian Journal of Animal Sciences* 27 (8): 1150–56.

16. "Alanine." n.d. Accessed March 31, 2021. https://aminoacidsguide.com/Ala.html.
17. Freibert. 2012. "ARGININE." April 21, 2012. https://aminoacidstudies.org/l-arginine/.
18. "Arginine." n.d. Accessed March 31, 2021. https://aminoacidsguide.com/Arg.html.
19. Carvalho, D. P., A. C. Ferreira, S. M. Coelho, J. M. Moraes, M. A. Camacho, and D. Rosenthal. 2000. "Thyroid Peroxidase Activity Is Inhibited by Amino Acids." *Brazilian Journal of Medical and Biological Research = Revista Brasileira de Pesquisas Medicas E Biologicas / Sociedade Brasileira de Biofisica... [et Al.]* 33 (3): 355–61.
20. Yamashita, Masatoshi, and Takanobu Yamamoto. 2014. "Tryptophan and Kynurenic Acid May Produce an Amplified Effect in Central Fatigue Induced by Chronic Sleep Disorder." *International Journal of Tryptophan Research: IJTR* 7 (May): 9–14.
21. Feksa, Luciane Rosa, Alexandra Latini, Virgínia Cielo Rech, Moacir Wajner, Carlos Severo Dutra-Filho, Angela Terezinha de Souza Wyse, and Clovis Milton Duval Wannmacher. 2006. "Promotion of Oxidative Stress by L-Tryptophan in Cerebral Cortex of Rats." *Neurochemistry International* 49 (1): 87–93.
22. Bertazzo, A., M. Biasiolo, C. V. Costa, E. Cardin de Stefani, and G. Allegri. 2000. "Tryptophan in Human Hair:

Correlation with Pigmentation." *Farmaco* 55 (8): 521–25.

23. Biasiolo, M., A. Bertazzo, C. V. Costa, and G. Allegri. 1999. "Correlation between Tryptophan and Hair Pigmentation in Human Hair." *Advances in Experimental Medicine and Biology* 467: 653–57.

24. Silber, B. Y., and J. A. J. Schmitt. 2010. "Effects of Tryptophan Loading on Human Cognition, Mood, and Sleep." *Neuroscience and Biobehavioral Reviews* 34 (3): 387–407.

25. Puka-Sundvall, M., P. Eriksson, M. Nilsson, M. Sandberg, and A. Lehmann. 1995. "Neurotoxicity of Cysteine: Interaction with Glutamate." *Brain Research* 705 (1–2): 65–70.

26. Viña, J., G. T. Saez, D. Wiggins, A. F. Roberts, R. Hems, and H. A. Krebs. 1983. "The Effect of Cysteine Oxidation on Isolated Hepatocytes." *Biochemical Journal* 212 (1): 39–44.

27. Janáky, R., V. Varga, A. Hermann, P. Saransaari, and S. S. Oja. 2000. "Mechanisms of L-Cysteine Neurotoxicity." *Neurochemical Research* 25 (9–10): 1397–1405.

28. Hayden, P. J., and J. L. Stevens. 1990. "Cysteine Conjugate Toxicity, Metabolism, and Binding to Macromolecules in Isolated Rat Kidney Mitochondria." *Molecular Pharmacology* 37 (3): 468–76.

29. Duranton, B., J. N. Freund, M. Galluser, R. Schleiffer, F. Gossé, C. Bergmann, M. Hasselmann, and F. Raul. 1999. "Promotion of Intestinal Carcinogenesis by Dietary Methionine." *Carcinogenesis* 20 (3): 493–97.

30. Yang, Yuhui, Jiahong Zhang, Guoqing Wu, Jin Sun, Yanan Wang, Haitao Guo, Yonghui Shi, Xiangrong Cheng, Xue

Tang, and Guowei Le. 2018. "Dietary Methionine Restriction Regulated Energy and Protein Homeostasis by Improving Thyroid Function in High Fat Diet Mice." *Food & Function* 9 (7): 3718–31.

31. "Health & Wellness Advocacy Studies - Clean Label Project." 2020. March 5, 2020. https://cleanlabelproject.org/health-fitness/.
32. Rossen, Jake. 2018. "Heavy Metal: Your Protein Powder May Contain Lead Or Arsenic." March 2, 2018. https://www.mentalfloss.com/article/533738/heavy-metal-your-protein-powder-may-contain-lead-or-arsenic.
33. "Health Risks of Protein Drinks - Consumer Reports." n.d. Accessed March 31, 2021. https://www.consumerreports.org/cro/2012/04/protein-drinks/index.htm.
34. https://althealthworks.com/15400/only-these-3-protein-powder-rated-free-of-lead-arsenic-and-mercury-popular-brands-failed-miserablyyelena/
35. Nordqvist, Joseph. 2017. "Whey Protein: Health Benefits, Side Effects, and Dangers." November 27, 2017. https://www.medicalnewstoday.com/articles/263371.
36. http://europepmc.org/article/med/18455389
37. Hulmi, Juha J., Jeff S. Volek, Harri Selänne, and Antti A. Mero. 2005. "Protein Ingestion prior to Strength Exercise Affects Blood Hormones and Metabolism." *Medicine and Science in Sports and Exercise* 37 (11): 1990–97.
38. Hulmi, Juha J., Jeff S. Volek, Harri Selänne, and Antti A. Mero. 2005. "Protein Ingestion prior to Strength Exercise Affects Blood Hormones and Metabolism." *Medicine and Science in Sports and Exercise* 37 (11): 1990–97.

39. Pape-Zambito, D. A., R. F. Roberts, and R. S. Kensinger. 2010. "Estrone and 17beta-Estradiol Concentrations in Pasteurized-Homogenized Milk and Commercial Dairy Products." *Journal of Dairy Science* 93 (6): 2533–40.

40. Ireland, Corydon. 2006. "Hormones in Milk Can Be Dangerous." Harvard Gazette. December 7, 2006. https://news.harvard.edu/gazette/story/2006/12/hormones-in-milk-can-be-dangerous/.

41. Farlow, Daniel W., Xia Xu, and Timothy D. Veenstra. 2009. "Quantitative Measurement of Endogenous Estrogen Metabolites, Risk-Factors for Development of Breast Cancer, in Commercial Milk Products by LC-MS/MS." *Journal of Chromatography. B, Analytical Technologies in the Biomedical and Life Sciences* 877 (13): 1327–34.

42. Zhu, Kun, Deborah A. Kerr, Xingqiong Meng, Amanda Devine, Vicky Solah, Colin W. Binns, and Richard L. Prince. 2015. "Two-Year Whey Protein Supplementation Did Not Enhance Muscle Mass and Physical Function in Well-Nourished Healthy Older Postmenopausal Women." *The Journal of Nutrition* 145 (11): 2520–26.

43. Hwang, Paul S., Thomas L. Andre, Sarah K. McKinley-Barnard, Flor E. Morales Marroquín, Joshua J. Gann, Joon J. Song, and Darryn S. Willoughby. 2017. "Resistance Training-Induced Elevations in Muscular Strength in Trained Men Are Maintained After 2 Weeks of Detraining and Not Differentially Affected by Whey Protein Supplementation." *Journal of Strength and Conditioning Research / National Strength & Conditioning Association* 31 (4): 869–81.

44. Boone, Carleigh H., Jeffrey R. Stout, Kyle S. Beyer,

David H. Fukuda, and Jay R. Hoffman. 2015. "Muscle Strength and Hypertrophy Occur Independently of Protein Supplementation during Short-Term Resistance Training in Untrained Men." *Applied Physiology, Nutrition, and Metabolism = Physiologie Appliquee, Nutrition et Metabolisme* 40 (8): 797–802.

45. Erskine, Robert M., Gareth Fletcher, Beth Hanson, and Jonathan P. Folland. 2012. "Whey Protein Does Not Enhance the Adaptations to Elbow Flexor Resistance Training." *Medicine and Science in Sports and Exercise* 44 (9): 1791–1800.
46. Weisgarber, Krissy D., Darren G. Candow, and Emelie S. M. Vogt. 2012. "Whey Protein before and during Resistance Exercise Has No Effect on Muscle Mass and Strength in Untrained Young Adults." *International Journal of Sport Nutrition and Exercise Metabolism* 22 (6): 463–69.
47. Mielke, Michelle, Terry J. Housh, Moh H. Malek, Travis W. Beck, Richard J. Schmidt, Glen O. Johnson, and Dona J. Housh. 2009. "The Effects of Whey Protein and Leucine Supplementation on Strength, Muscular Endurance, and Body Composition during Resistance Training." *Journal of Exercise Physiology Online / American Society of Exercise Physiologists* 12 (5): 39–50.
48. Verdijk, Lex B., Richard A. M. Jonkers, Benjamin G. Gleeson, Milou Beelen, Kenneth Meijer, Hans H. C. M. Savelberg, Will K. W. H. Wodzig, Paul Dendale, and Luc J. C. van Loon. 2009. "Protein Supplementation before and after Exercise Does Not Further Augment Skeletal Muscle Hypertrophy after Resistance Training in Elderly Men." *The American Journal of Clinical Nutrition* 89 (2): 608–16.

49. Melnik, B. C. 2011. "Evidence for Acne-Promoting Effects of Milk and Other Insulinotropic Dairy Products." In , 67:131–45.

50. Silverberg, Nanette B. 2012. "Whey Protein Precipitating Moderate to Severe Acne Flares in 5 Teenaged Athletes." *Cutis; Cutaneous Medicine for the Practitioner* 90 (2): 70–72.

51. Pontes, Thaís de Carvalho, Gilson Mauro Costa Fernandes Filho, Arthur de Sousa Pereira Trindade, and Jader Freire Sobral Filho. 2013. "Incidence of Acne Vulgaris in Young Adult Users of Protein-Calorie Supplements in the City of João Pessoa--PB." *Anais Brasileiros de Dermatologia* 88 (6): 907–12.

52. Simonart, Thierry. 2012. "Acne and Whey Protein Supplementation among Bodybuilders." *Dermatology* 225 (3): 256–58.

53. Adebamowo, Clement A., Donna Spiegelman, F. William Danby, A. Lindsay Frazier, Walter C. Willett, and Michelle D. Holmes. 2005. "High School Dietary Dairy Intake and Teenage Acne." *Journal of the American Academy of Dermatology* 52 (2): 207–14.

54. Bowen, Jane, Manny Noakes, Craige Trenerry, and Peter M. Clifton. 2006. "Energy Intake, Ghrelin, and Cholecystokinin after Different Carbohydrate and Protein Preloads in Overweight Men." *The Journal of Clinical Endocrinology and Metabolism* 91 (4): 1477–83.

55. Bellissimo, N., M. V. Desantadina, P. B. Pencharz, G. B. Berall, S. G. Thomas, and G. H. Anderson. 2008. "A Comparison of Short-Term Appetite and Energy Intakes in Normal Weight and Obese Boys Following Glucose and

Whey-Protein Drinks." *International Journal of Obesity* 32 (2): 362–71.

56. Aldrich, Noel D., Marla M. Reicks, Shalamar D. Sibley, J. Bruce Redmon, William Thomas, and Susan K. Raatz. 2011. "Varying Protein Source and Quantity Do Not Significantly Improve Weight Loss, Fat Loss, or Satiety in Reduced Energy Diets among Midlife Adults." *Nutrition Research* 31 (2): 104–12.
57. Abou-Samra, Rania, Lian Keersmaekers, Dino Brienza, Rajat Mukherjee, and Katherine Macé. 2011. "Effect of Different Protein Sources on Satiation and Short-Term Satiety When Consumed as a Starter." *Nutrition Journal* 10 (December): 139.
58. Arnberg, Karina, Christian Mølgaard, Kim Fleischer Michaelsen, Signe Marie Jensen, Ellen Trolle, and Anni Larnkjær. 2012. "Skim Milk, Whey, and Casein Increase Body Weight and Whey and Casein Increase the Plasma C-Peptide Concentration in Overweight Adolescents." *The Journal of Nutrition* 142 (12): 2083–90.
59. Hoppe, C., C. Mølgaard, A. Vaag, V. Barkholt, and K. F. Michaelsen. 2005. "High Intakes of Milk, but Not Meat, Increase S-Insulin and Insulin Resistance in 8-Year-Old Boys." *European Journal of Clinical Nutrition* 59 (3): 393–98.
60. Liljeberg Elmståhl, H., and I. Björck. 2001. "Milk as a Supplement to Mixed Meals May Elevate Postprandial Insulinaemia." *European Journal of Clinical Nutrition* 55 (11): 994–99.
61. Melnik, B. C. 2011. "Evidence for Acne-Promoting Effects of Milk and Other Insulinotropic Dairy Products." In ,

67:131–45.

62. Habib, Huma, and K. M. Fazili. 2007. "Plant Protease Inhibitors: A Defense Strategy in Plants." https://www.semanticscholar.org/paper/bd43c4f85fd90214638535119278ad31597a7436.

63. "Proteins." 2015. May 10, 2015. https://basicbiology.net/micro/biochemistry/protein.

64. "What Are Proteins and What Do They Do?" n.d. Accessed March 31, 2021. https://medlineplus.gov/genetics/understanding/howgeneswork/protein/.

65. "The Protein Bible: Part 3 - Protein Requirements for Goals." n.d. Accessed March 31, 2021. http://www.schwarzenegger.com/fitness/post/The-Protein-Bible-Part-3-Protein-Requirements-for-Goals.

66. Evans, William J. 2004. "Protein Nutrition, Exercise and Aging." *Journal of the American College of Nutrition* 23 (6 Suppl): 601S - 609S.

67. Campbell, W. W., T. A. Trappe, R. R. Wolfe, and W. J. Evans. 2001. "The Recommended Dietary Allowance for Protein May Not Be Adequate for Older People to Maintain Skeletal Muscle." *The Journals of Gerontology. Series A, Biological Sciences and Medical Sciences* 56 (6): M373–80.

68. Lonnie, Marta, Emma Hooker, Jeffrey M. Brunstrom, Bernard M. Corfe, Mark A. Green, Anthony W. Watson, Elizabeth A. Williams, Emma J. Stevenson, Simon Penson, and Alexandra M. Johnstone. 2018. "Protein for Life: Review of Optimal Protein Intake, Sustainable Dietary Sources and the Effect on Appetite in Ageing Adults." *Nutrients* 10 (3). https://doi.org/10.3390/nu10030360.

69. Witard, Oliver C., Sophie L. Wardle, Lindsay S. Macnaughton, Adrian B. Hodgson, and Kevin D. Tipton. 2016. "Protein Considerations for Optimising Skeletal Muscle Mass in Healthy Young and Older Adults." *Nutrients* 8 (4): 181.

70. Smith, J. S., C. B. Brachmann, I. Celic, M. A. Kenna, S. Muhammad, V. J. Starai, J. L. Avalos, et al. 2000. "A Phylogenetically Conserved NAD+-Dependent Protein Deacetylase Activity in the Sir2 Protein Family." *Proceedings of the National Academy of Sciences of the United States of America* 97 (12): 6658–63.

71. Seyedsadjadi, Neda, Jade Berg, Ayse A. Bilgin, Nady Braidy, Chris Salonikas, and Ross Grant. 2018. "High Protein Intake Is Associated with Low Plasma NAD+ Levels in a Healthy Human Cohort." *PloS One* 13 (8): e0201968.

Chapter 6 - Vegetables

1. Wright, E. 1958. "Goitrogen of Milk Produced on Kale." *Nature* 181 (4623): 1602–3.

2. http://whqlibdoc.who.int/cgi-bin/repository.pl?url=/bulletin/1968/Vol38/Vol38-No2/bulletin_1968_38(2)_297-318.pdf

3. Smith, R. H. 1978. "S-Methylcysteine Sulphoxide, the Brassica Anaemia Factor (a Valuable Dietary Factor for Man?)." *Veterinary Science Communications* 2 (1): 47–61.

4. Davies, M. H., J. M. Ngong, A. Pean, C. R. Vickers, R. H. Waring, and E. Elias. 1995. "Sulphoxidation and Sulphation Capacity in Patients with Primary Biliary Cirrhosis." *Journal of Hepatology* 22 (5): 551–60.

5. Gordon, C., H. Bradley, R. H. Waring, and P. Emery. 1992. "Abnormal Sulphur Oxidation in Systemic Lupus Erythematosus." *The Lancet* 339 (8784): 25–26.
6. Emery, P., H. Bradley, V. Arthur, E. Tunn, and R. Waring. 1992. "Genetic Factors Influencing the Outcome of Early Arthritis--the Role of Sulphoxidation Status." *British Journal of Rheumatology* 31 (7): 449–51.
7. Chris Kresser, M. S. 2012. "Myths and Truths About Fiber." Chris Kresser LLC. February 17, 2012. https://chriskresser.com/myths-and-truths-about-fiber/.
8. Gillespie, David. n.d. "4 Good Reasons Not to Add Fibre to Your Diet." Accessed April 1, 2021. https://davidgillespie.org/4-good-reasons-not-to-add-fibre-to-your-diet/.
9. Greenfield, Ben. 2013. "Is Fiber Bad For You?" January 12, 2013. https://bengreenfieldfitness.com/article/nutrition-articles/is-fiber-bad-for-you/.
10. Guest. 2013. "Dietary Fiber Is Bad for Sex - That's the Only Claim About It That Isn't a Myth." September 3, 2013. https://www.marksdailyapple.com/dietary-fiber-is-bad-for-sex-thats-the-only-claim-about-it-that-isnt-a-myth/.
11. Wanders, A. J., J. J. G. C. van den Borne, C. de Graaf, T. Hulshof, M. C. Jonathan, M. Kristensen, M. Mars, H. A. Schols, and E. J. M. Feskens. 2011. "Effects of Dietary Fibre on Subjective Appetite, Energy Intake and Body Weight: A Systematic Review of Randomized Controlled Trials." *Obesity Reviews: An Official Journal of the International Association for the Study of Obesity* 12 (9): 724–39.
12. Clark, Michelle J., and Joanne L. Slavin. 2013. "The Effect

of Fiber on Satiety and Food Intake: A Systematic Review." *Journal of the American College of Nutrition* 32 (3): 200–211.

13. Clark, Michelle J., and Joanne L. Slavin. 2013. "The Effect of Fiber on Satiety and Food Intake: A Systematic Review." *Journal of the American College of Nutrition* 32 (3): 200–211.
14. Asano, T., and R. S. McLeod. 2002. "Dietary Fibre for the Prevention of Colorectal Adenomas and Carcinomas." *Cochrane Database of Systematic Reviews*, no. 2: CD003430.
15. Park, Yikyung, David J. Hunter, Donna Spiegelman, Leif Bergkvist, Franco Berrino, Piet A. van den Brandt, Julie E. Buring, et al. 2005. "Dietary Fiber Intake and Risk of Colorectal Cancer: A Pooled Analysis of Prospective Cohort Studies." *JAMA: The Journal of the American Medical Association* 294 (22): 2849–57.
16. Alberts, D. S., M. E. Martínez, D. J. Roe, J. M. Guillén-Rodríguez, J. R. Marshall, J. B. van Leeuwen, M. E. Reid, et al. 2000. "Lack of Effect of a High-Fiber Cereal Supplement on the Recurrence of Colorectal Adenomas. Phoenix Colon Cancer Prevention Physicians' Network." *The New England Journal of Medicine* 342 (16): 1156–62.
17. Jacobs, Elizabeth T., Anna R. Giuliano, Denise J. Roe, José M. Guillén-Rodríguez, Lisa M. Hess, David S. Alberts, and María Elena Martínez. 2002. "Intake of Supplemental and Total Fiber and Risk of Colorectal Adenoma Recurrence in the Wheat Bran Fiber Trial." *Cancer Epidemiology, Biomarkers & Prevention: A Publication of the American Association for Cancer Research, Cosponsored by the American Society of Preventive Oncology* 11 (9): 906–14.
18. Jacobs, Elizabeth T., Anna R. Giuliano, Denise J. Roe, José

M. Guillén-Rodríguez, David S. Alberts, and María Elena Martínez. 2002. "Baseline Dietary Fiber Intake and Colorectal Adenoma Recurrence in the Wheat Bran Fiber Randomized Trial." *Journal of the National Cancer Institute* 94 (21): 1620–25.

19. Ho, Kok-Sun, Charmaine You Mei Tan, Muhd Ashik Mohd Daud, and Francis Seow-Choen. 2012. "Stopping or Reducing Dietary Fiber Intake Reduces Constipation and Its Associated Symptoms." *World Journal of Gastroenterology: WJG* 18 (33): 4593–96.
20. Bijkerk, C. J., J. W. M. Muris, J. A. Knottnerus, A. W. Hoes, and N. J. de Wit. 2004. "Systematic Review: The Role of Different Types of Fibre in the Treatment of Irritable Bowel Syndrome." *Alimentary Pharmacology & Therapeutics* 19 (3): 245–51.
21. Peery, Anne F., Patrick R. Barrett, Doyun Park, Albert J. Rogers, Joseph A. Galanko, Christopher F. Martin, and Robert S. Sandler. 2012. "A High-Fiber Diet Does Not Protect against Asymptomatic Diverticulosis." *Gastroenterology* 142 (2): 266–72.e1.
22. Carvalho, Erica Bloes de, Márcia Regina Vitolo, Cíntia Mendes Gama, Fabio Ancona Lopez, José Augusto C. Taddei, and Mauro Batista de Morais. 2006. "Fiber Intake, Constipation, and Overweight among Adolescents Living in Sao Paulo City." *Nutrition* 22 (7–8): 744–49.
23. "Fiber." n.d. Accessed April 1, 2021. https://medlineplus.gov/ency/article/002470.htm.
24. "Soluble vs. Insoluble Fiber." n.d. Accessed April 1, 2021. https://medlineplus.gov/ency/article/002136.htm.

25. Vineetha. n.d. "Traditional Asian Diet - What Is It, Dietary Guidelines & A Simple Diet Chart - Health Beckon." Accessed April 1, 2021. https://www.healthbeckon.com/traditional-asian-diet/.

26. Administrator, G. I. Care. 2011. "Asian Diet." October 29, 2011. https://www.gicare.com/gi-health-resources/asian-diet/.

27. Wu, A. H., A. S. Whittemore, L. N. Kolonel, E. M. John, R. P. Gallagher, D. W. West, J. Hankin, C. Z. Teh, D. M. Dreon, and R. S. Paffenbarger Jr. 1995. "Serum Androgens and Sex Hormone-Binding Globulins in Relation to Lifestyle Factors in Older African-American, White, and Asian Men in the United States and Canada." *Cancer Epidemiology, Biomarkers & Prevention: A Publication of the American Association for Cancer Research, Cosponsored by the American Society of Preventive Oncology* 4 (7): 735–41.

28. Whitten, Crystal G., and Terry D. Shultz. 1988. "Binding of Steroid Hormones in Vitro by Water-Insoluble Dietary Fiber." *Nutrition Research* 8 (11): 1223–35.

29. Ross, J. K., D. J. Pusateri, and T. D. Shultz. 1990. "Dietary and Hormonal Evaluation of Men at Different Risks for Prostate Cancer: Fiber Intake, Excretion, and Composition, with in Vitro Evidence for an Association between Steroid Hormones and Specific Fiber Components." *The American Journal of Clinical Nutrition* 51 (3): 365–70.

30. Dorgan, J. F., J. T. Judd, C. Longcope, C. Brown, A. Schatzkin, B. A. Clevidence, W. S. Campbell, et al. 1996. "Effects of Dietary Fat and Fiber on Plasma and Urine Androgens and Estrogens in Men: A Controlled Feeding

Study." *The American Journal of Clinical Nutrition* 64 (6): 850–55.

31. Wang, Christina, Don H. Catlin, Borislav Starcevic, David Heber, Christie Ambler, Nancy Berman, Geraldine Lucas, et al. 2005. "Low-Fat High-Fiber Diet Decreased Serum and Urine Androgens in Men." *The Journal of Clinical Endocrinology and Metabolism* 90 (6): 3550–59.
32. Shultz, T. D., and B. J. Howie. 1986. "In Vitro Binding of Steroid Hormones by Natural and Purified Fibers." *Nutrition and Cancer* 8 (2): 141–47.
33. Field, A. E., G. A. Colditz, W. C. Willett, C. Longcope, and J. B. McKinlay. 1994. "The Relation of Smoking, Age, Relative Weight, and Dietary Intake to Serum Adrenal Steroids, Sex Hormones, and Sex Hormone-Binding Globulin in Middle-Aged Men." *The Journal of Clinical Endocrinology and Metabolism* 79 (5): 1310–16.
34. Herman Adlercreutz (1990) Western diet and Western diseases: Some hormonal and biochemical mechanisms and associations, Scandinavian Journal of Clinical and Laboratory Investigation, 50:sup201, 3-23, DOI: 10.1080/00365519009085798
35. http://www.airlats.com/testosterone/
36. Tymchuk, C. N., S. B. Tessler, and R. J. Barnard. 2000. "Changes in Sex Hormone-Binding Globulin, Insulin, and Serum Lipids in Postmenopausal Women on a Low-Fat, High-Fiber Diet Combined with Exercise." *Nutrition and Cancer* 38 (2): 158–62.
37. "Gas – Flatulence: MedlinePlus Medical Encyclopedia." n.d. Accessed April 1, 2021. https://medlineplus.gov/ency/

article/003124.htm.

38. Torre, M., A. R. Rodriguez, and F. Saura-Calixto. 1991. "Effects of Dietary Fiber and Phytic Acid on Mineral Availability." *Critical Reviews in Food Science and Nutrition* 30 (1): 1–22.

39. Weickert, Martin O., and Andreas F. H. Pfeiffer. 2008. "Metabolic Effects of Dietary Fiber Consumption and Prevention of Diabetes." *The Journal of Nutrition* 138 (3): 439–42.

40. Weickert, Martin O., and Andreas F. H. Pfeiffer. 2018. "Impact of Dietary Fiber Consumption on Insulin Resistance and the Prevention of Type 2 Diabetes." *The Journal of Nutrition* 148 (1): 7–12.

41. Higgins, Janine A. 2004. "Resistant Starch: Metabolic Effects and Potential Health Benefits." *Journal of AOAC International* 87 (3): 761–68.

42. Robertson, M. Denise, Alex S. Bickerton, A. Louise Dennis, Hubert Vidal, and Keith N. Frayn. 2005. "Insulin-Sensitizing Effects of Dietary Resistant Starch and Effects on Skeletal Muscle and Adipose Tissue Metabolism." *The American Journal of Clinical Nutrition* 82 (3): 559–67.

43. Roos, N. de, M. L. Heijnen, C. de Graaf, G. Woestenenk, and E. Hobbel. 1995. "Resistant Starch Has Little Effect on Appetite, Food Intake and Insulin Secretion of Healthy Young Men." *European Journal of Clinical Nutrition* 49 (7): 532–41.

44. Polakof, Sergio, María Elena Díaz-Rubio, Dominique Dardevet, Jean-François Martin, Estelle Pujos-Guillot, Augustin Scalbert, Jean-Louis Sebedio, Andrzej Mazur, and Blandine Comte. 2013. "Resistant Starch Intake Partly

Restores Metabolic and Inflammatory Alterations in the Liver of High-Fat-Diet-Fed Rats." *The Journal of Nutritional Biochemistry* 24 (11): 1920–30.

45. Li, Qian, Theodore R. Holford, Yawei Zhang, Peter Boyle, Susan T. Mayne, Min Dai, and Tongzhang Zheng. 2013. "Dietary Fiber Intake and Risk of Breast Cancer by Menopausal and Estrogen Receptor Status." *European Journal of Nutrition* 52 (1): 217–23.

46. Parnell, Jill A., and Raylene A. Reimer. 2009. "Weight Loss during Oligofructose Supplementation Is Associated with Decreased Ghrelin and Increased Peptide YY in Overweight and Obese Adults." *The American Journal of Clinical Nutrition* 89 (6): 1751–59.

47. Kok, N., M. Roberfroid, and N. Delzenne. 1996. "Dietary Oligofructose Modifies the Impact of Fructose on Hepatic Triacylglycerol Metabolism." *Metabolism: Clinical and Experimental* 45 (12): 1547–50.

48. Cashman, Kevin D. 2006. "A Prebiotic Substance Persistently Enhances Intestinal Calcium Absorption and Increases Bone Mineralization in Young Adolescents." *Nutrition Reviews* 64 (4): 189–96.

49. Guarner, Francisco. 2007. "Studies with Inulin-Type Fructans on Intestinal Infections, Permeability, and Inflammation." *The Journal of Nutrition* 137 (11 Suppl): 2568S – 2571S.

50. Guarner, Francisco, and Juan-R Malagelada. 2003. "Gut Flora in Health and Disease." *The Lancet* 361 (9356): 512–19.

51. Roberfroid, M. 1993. "Dietary Fiber, Inulin, and Oligofructose: A Review Comparing Their Physiological

Effects." *Critical Reviews in Food Science and Nutrition* 33 (2): 103–48.

52. Arslanoglu, Sertac, Guido E. Moro, Joachim Schmitt, Laura Tandoi, Silvia Rizzardi, and Gunther Boehm. 2008. "Early Dietary Intervention with a Mixture of Prebiotic Oligosaccharides Reduces the Incidence of Allergic Manifestations and Infections during the First Two Years of Life." *The Journal of Nutrition* 138 (6): 1091–95.
53. Guarner, Francisco. 2007. "Studies with Inulin-Type Fructans on Intestinal Infections, Permeability, and Inflammation." *The Journal of Nutrition* 137 (11 Suppl): 2568S - 2571S.

Chapter 7 - Hormones

1. Fountain, John H., and Sarah L. Lappin. 2020. "Physiology, Renin Angiotensin System." In *StatPearls*. Treasure Island (FL): StatPearls Publishing.
2. Tuso, Phillip. 2014. "Prediabetes and Lifestyle Modification: Time to Prevent a Preventable Disease." *The Permanente Journal* 18 (3): 88–93.

Chapter 8 - Inflammation

1. Peat, Ray. n.d. "Regeneration and Degeneration." Accessed April 1, 2021. https://raypeat.com/articles/articles/regeneration-degeneration.shtml.
2. Zamenhof, S., and G. Ahmad. 1979. "The Effects of Exogenous Nutrients on Growth of Chick Embryo Brain."

Growth 43 (3): 160–66.

3. https://web.stanford.edu/group/stanfordbirds/text/essays/Precocial_and_Altricial.html
4. Rinaldi, Joshua. 2006. "Last caw: Crow thought to be world's oldest dies in Bearsville at age 59." July 7, 2006. https://www.dailyfreeman.com/news/last-caw-crow-thought-to-be-world-s-oldest-dies/article_985aeacb-4ea2-5ea4-8cce-1e7037763e5b.html.
5. "UCSB Science Line." n.d. Accessed April 1, 2021. http://scienceline.ucsb.edu/getkey.php?key=6040.
6. Wojdasiewicz, Piotr, Łukasz A. Poniatowski, and Dariusz Szukiewicz. 2014. "The Role of Inflammatory and Anti-Inflammatory Cytokines in the Pathogenesis of Osteoarthritis." *Mediators of Inflammation* 2014 (April): 561459.
7. Wagner, W., and M. Wehrmann. 2007. "Differential Cytokine Activity and Morphology during Wound Healing in the Neonatal and Adult Rat Skin." *Journal of Cellular and Molecular Medicine* 11 (6): 1342–51.
8. Morykwas, M. J., S. L. Perry, and L. C. Argenta. 1993. "Effects of Prostaglandins and Indomethacin on the Cellular Inflammatory Response Following Surgical Trauma in Fetal Rabbits." *International Journal of Tissue Reactions* 15 (4): 151–56.
9. Ricciotti, Emanuela, and Garret A. FitzGerald. 2011. "Prostaglandins and Inflammation." *Arteriosclerosis, Thrombosis, and Vascular Biology* 31 (5): 986–1000.
10. Dirix, Chantal E. H., Arnold D. Kester, and Gerard Hornstra. 2009. "Associations between Term Birth

Dimensions and Prenatal Exposure to Essential and Trans Fatty Acids." *Early Human Development* 85 (8): 525–30.

11. Dirix, C. E. H., G. Hornstra, and J. G. Nijhuis. 2009. "Fetal Learning and Memory: Weak Associations with the Early Essential Polyunsaturated Fatty Acid Status." *Prostaglandins, Leukotrienes, and Essential Fatty Acids* 80 (4): 207–12.

12. Sweeney, B., P. Puri, and D. J. Reen. 2001. "Polyunsaturated Fatty Acids Influence Neonatal Monocyte Survival." *Pediatric Surgery International* 17 (4): 254–58.

13. Kent, George. 2014. "Regulating Fatty Acids in Infant Formula: Critical Assessment of U.S. Policies and Practices." *International Breastfeeding Journal* 9 (1): 2.

14. Peltekova, Vanya, Doreen Engelberts, Gail Otulakowski, Satoko Uematsu, Martin Post, and Brian P. Kavanagh. 2010. "Hypercapnic Acidosis in Ventilator-Induced Lung Injury." *Intensive Care Medicine* 36 (5): 869–78.

15. Peng, Yuanfei, Minhua Zheng, Qing Ye, Xuehua Chen, Beiqing Yu, and Bingya Liu. 2009. "Heated and Humidified CO2 Prevents Hypothermia, Peritoneal Injury, and Intra-Abdominal Adhesions during Prolonged Laparoscopic Insufflations." *The Journal of Surgical Research* 151 (1): 40–47.

16. Peng, Yuanfei, Minhua Zheng, Qing Ye, Xuehua Chen, Beiqing Yu, and Bingya Liu. 2009. "Heated and Humidified CO2 Prevents Hypothermia, Peritoneal Injury, and Intra-Abdominal Adhesions during Prolonged Laparoscopic Insufflations." *The Journal of Surgical Research* 151 (1): 40–47.

17. Morisaki, Hiroshi, Satoshi Yajima, Yoko Watanabe, Takeshi Suzuki, Michiko Yamamoto, Nobuyuki Katori, Saori Hashiguchi, and Junzo Takeda. 2009. "Hypercapnic Acidosis

Minimizes Endotoxin-Induced Gut Mucosal Injury in Rabbits." *Intensive Care Medicine* 35 (1): 129–35.

18. Grow, Matthew, Anton W. Neff, Anthony L. Mescher, and Michael W. King. 2006. "Global Analysis of Gene Expression in Xenopus Hindlimbs during Stage-Dependent Complete and Incomplete Regeneration." *Developmental Dynamics: An Official Publication of the American Association of Anatomists* 235 (10): 2667–85.
19. Winkelmann, E. 1960. "[Experimental studies on the regeneration of the spinal cord of Amblystoma mexicanum after extirpation of a small section]." *Zeitschrift fur mikroskopisch-anatomische Forschung* 66: 147–76.
20. Shieh, Shyh-Jou, and Tsun-Chih Cheng. 2015. "Regeneration and Repair of Human Digits and Limbs: Fact and Fiction." *Regeneration (Oxford, England)* 2 (4): 149–68.
21. Jafari, Paris, Camillo Muller, Anthony Grognuz, Lee Ann Applegate, Wassim Raffoul, Pietro G. di Summa, and Sébastien Durand. 2017. "First Insights into Human Fingertip Regeneration by Echo-Doppler Imaging and Wound Microenvironment Assessment." *International Journal of Molecular Sciences* 18 (5). https://doi.org/10.3390/ijms18051054.
22. Mescher, Anthony L., Anton W. Neff, and Michael W. King. 2017. "Inflammation and Immunity in Organ Regeneration." *Developmental and Comparative Immunology* 66 (January): 98–110.
23. Elmore, Susan. 2007. "Apoptosis: A Review of Programmed Cell Death." *Toxicologic Pathology* 35 (4): 495–516.

24. Kurata, Y., Y. Nishioeda, T. Tsubakio, and T. Kitani. 1980. "Thrombocytopenia in Graves' Disease: Effect of T3 on Platelet Kinetics." *Acta Haematologica* 63 (4): 185–90.

25. Aprahamian, T., Y. Takemura, D. Goukassian, and K. Walsh. 2008. "Ageing Is Associated with Diminished Apoptotic Cell Clearance in Vivo." *Clinical and Experimental Immunology* 152 (3): 448–55.

26. Aprahamian, T., Y. Takemura, D. Goukassian, and K. Walsh. 2008. "Ageing Is Associated with Diminished Apoptotic Cell Clearance in Vivo." *Clinical and Experimental Immunology* 152 (3): 448–55.

27. Zhong, Zhi, Micheal D. Wheeler, Xiangli Li, Matthias Froh, Peter Schemmer, Ming Yin, Hartwig Bunzendaul, Blair Bradford, and John J. Lemasters. 2003. "L-Glycine: A Novel Antiinflammatory, Immunomodulatory, and Cytoprotective Agent." *Current Opinion in Clinical Nutrition and Metabolic Care* 6 (2): 229–40.

28. Purves, Dale, George J. Augustine, David Fitzpatrick, Lawrence C. Katz, Anthony-Samuel LaMantia, James O. McNamara, and S. Mark Williams. 2001. *GABA and Glycine*. Sinauer Associates.

29. Lynch, Joseph W. 2004. "Molecular Structure and Function of the Glycine Receptor Chloride Channel." *Physiological Reviews* 84 (4): 1051–95.

30. Van den Eynden, Jimmy, Sheen Saheb Ali, Nikki Horwood, Sofie Carmans, Bert Brône, Niels Hellings, Paul Steels, Robert J. Harvey, and Jean-Michel Rigo. 2009. "Glycine and Glycine Receptor Signalling in Non-Neuronal Cells." *Frontiers in Molecular Neuroscience* 2 (August): 9.

31. (Valtsu), Vladimir Heiskanen, and View my Complete Profile. n.d. "Valtsu's." Accessed April 1, 2021. https://valtsus.blogspot.com/2013/12/glycine.html.

32. Stone, Matt. 2014. "Diet and Inflammation Part 4 - 180 Degree Health." September 20, 2014. https://180degreehealth.com/diet-inflammation-part-4/.

33. Comp Biochem Physiol C Toxicol Pharmacol. 2003 Apr;134(4):521-7. **Effect of glycine in streptozotocin-induced diabetic rats.** Alvarado-Vásquez N, Zamudio P, Cerón E, Vanda B, Zenteno E, Carvajal-Sandoval G.

34. Mol Vis. 2012;18:439-48. **Glycine therapy inhibits the progression of cataract in streptozotocin-induced diabetic rats.** Bahmani F, Bathaie SZ, Aldavood SJ, Ghahghaei A.

35. Rev Alerg Mex. 2006 Nov-Dec;53(6):212-6. **Effect of glycine on the immune response of the experimentally diabetic rats.** Lezcano Meza D, Terán Ortiz L, Carvajal Sandoval G, Gutiérrez de la Cadena M, Terán Escandón D, Estrada Parra S.

36. Rev Med Chil. 2010 Oct;138(10):1246-52. **[Effects of glycine on auditory evoked potentials among diabetic patients with auditory pathway neuropathy].** [Article in Spanish] Muñoz-Carlin Mde L, Rodríguez-Moctezuma JR, Gómez Latorre JG, Montes-Castillo ML, Juárez-Adauta S.

37. Life Sci. 2006 Jun 13;79(3):225-32. **Oral glycine administration attenuates diabetic complications in streptozotocin-induced diabetic rats.** Alvarado-Vásquez N, Lascurain R, Cerón E, Vanda B, Carvajal-Sandoval G, Tapia A, Guevara J, Montaño LF, Zenteno E.

38. Journal of Kerman University of Medical Sciences

2014;21 **Assessment of Oral Glycine and Lysine Therapy on Receptor for Advanced Glycation End Products and Transforming Growth Factor Beta Expression in the Kidney of Streptozotocin-Induced Diabetic Rats in Comparison with Normal Rats.** Somayeh Sadat Heidary, M.Sc., et al.

39. Journal of Experimental & Clinical Medicine 2013;5:109-114 **Effect of Glycine on Protein Oxidation and Advanced Glycation End Products Formation** Salinas Arreortua Noe, García Lorenzana Mario, Genoveva Durán Reyes, Villagómez Jasso Edgar Iván, Alarcón Aguilar Francisco Javier, Gómez Olivares José Luis "The experimental data demonstrate that glycine reduced glucose, HbA1C, and fructosamine levels in blood. Even more, glycine significantly reduced AGE-BSA conformation, but the reduction of protein oxidation occurred only in the kidneys."

40. Carcinogenesis. 1999 Nov;20(11):2075-81. **Dietary glycine prevents the development of liver tumors caused by the peroxisome proliferator WY-14,643.** Rose ML, Cattley RC, Dunn C, Wong V, Li X, Thurman RG.

41. "Turmeric." n.d. Accessed April 1, 2021. https://www.nccih.nih.gov/health/turmeric.

42. Kuptniratsaikul, Vilai, Sunee Thanakhumtorn, Pornsiri Chinswangwatanakul, Luksamee Wattanamongkonsil, and Visanu Thamlikitkul. 2009. "Efficacy and Safety of Curcuma Domestica Extracts in Patients with Knee Osteoarthritis." *Journal of Alternative and Complementary Medicine* 15 (8): 891–97.

43. Daily, James W., Mini Yang, and Sunmin Park. 2016. "Efficacy of Turmeric Extracts and Curcumin for Alleviating

the Symptoms of Joint Arthritis: A Systematic Review and Meta-Analysis of Randomized Clinical Trials." *Journal of Medicinal Food* 19 (8): 717–29.

44. "Supplement and Herb Guide for Arthritis Symptoms." n.d. Accessed April 1, 2021. https://www.arthritis.org/health-wellness/treatment/complementary-therapies/supplements-and-vitamins/supplement-and-herb-guide-for-arthritis-symptoms.

45. Kim, Dong-Chan, Sae-Kwang Ku, and Jong-Sup Bae. 2012. "Anticoagulant Activities of Curcumin and Its Derivative." *BMB Reports* 45 (4): 221–26.

46. Kulkarni, S. K., and A. Dhir. 2010. "An Overview of Curcumin in Neurological Disorders." *Indian Journal of Pharmaceutical Sciences* 72 (2): 149–54.

47. Kathleen Jade, N. D. 2019. "2 Natural Antidepressants Found to Be as Effective as Prozac - University Health News." March 21, 2019. https://universityhealthnews.com/daily/depression/2-natural-antidepressants-found-to-be-as-effective-as-prozac/.

48. Yu, Jing-Jie, Liu-Bao Pei, Yong Zhang, Zi-Yu Wen, and Jian-Li Yang. 2015. "Chronic Supplementation of Curcumin Enhances the Efficacy of Antidepressants in Major Depressive Disorder: A Randomized, Double-Blind, Placebo-Controlled Pilot Study." *Journal of Clinical Psychopharmacology* 35 (4): 406–10.

49. Akinyemi, Ayodele Jacob, Gustavo Roberto Thomé, Vera Maria Morsch, Nathieli B. Bottari, Jucimara Baldissarelli, Lizielle Souza de Oliveira, Jeferson Ferraz Goularte, et al. 2016. "Effect of Ginger and Turmeric Rhizomes on

Inflammatory Cytokines Levels and Enzyme Activities of Cholinergic and Purinergic Systems in Hypertensive Rats." *Planta Medica* 82 (7): 612–20.

50. Charles, V., and S. X. Charles. 1992. "The Use and Efficacy of Azadirachta Indica ADR ('Neem') and Curcuma Longa ('Turmeric') in Scabies. A Pilot Study." *Tropical and Geographical Medicine* 44 (1–2): 178–81.

51. Siddiqui, M. Z. 2011. "Boswellia Serrata, a Potential Antiinflammatory Agent: An Overview." *Indian Journal of Pharmaceutical Sciences* 73 (3): 255–61.

52. Su, Shulan, Jinao Duan, Ting Chen, Xiaochen Huang, Erxin Shang, Li Yu, Kaifeng Wei, et al. 2015. "Frankincense and Myrrh Suppress Inflammation via Regulation of the Metabolic Profiling and the MAPK Signaling Pathway." *Scientific Reports* 5 (September): 13668.

53. Ernst, E. 2008. "Frankincense: Systematic Review." *BMJ* 337 (December): a2813.

54. Blain, Emma J., Ahmed Y. Ali, and Victor C. Duance. 2010. "Boswellia Frereana (frankincense) Suppresses Cytokine-Induced Matrix Metalloproteinase Expression and Production of pro-Inflammatory Molecules in Articular Cartilage." *Phytotherapy Research: PTR* 24 (6): 905–12.

55. Blain, Emma J., Ahmed Y. Ali, and Victor C. Duance. 2010. "Boswellia Frereana (frankincense) Suppresses Cytokine-Induced Matrix Metalloproteinase Expression and Production of pro-Inflammatory Molecules in Articular Cartilage." *Phytotherapy Research: PTR* 24 (6): 905–12.

56. Straube, Sebastian, Martin R. Tramèr, R. Andrew Moore, Sheena Derry, and Henry J. McQuay. 2009. "Mortality with

Upper Gastrointestinal Bleeding and Perforation: Effects of Time and NSAID Use." *BMC Gastroenterology* 9 (June): 41.

57. Straube, Sebastian, Martin R. Tramèr, R. Andrew Moore, Sheena Derry, and Henry J. McQuay. 2009. "Mortality with Upper Gastrointestinal Bleeding and Perforation: Effects of Time and NSAID Use." *BMC Gastroenterology* 9 (June): 41.

58. Roxas, Mario. 2008. "The Role of Enzyme Supplementation in Digestive Disorders." Alternative Medicine Review: *A Journal of Clinical Therapeutic* 13 (4): 307–14.

59. Kerkhoffs, G. M. M. J., P. A. A. Struijs, C. de Wit, V. W. Rahlfs, H. Zwipp, and C. N. van Dijk. 2004. "A Double Blind, Randomised, Parallel Group Study on the Efficacy and Safety of Treating Acute Lateral Ankle Sprain with Oral Hydrolytic Enzymes." *British Journal of Sports Medicine* 38 (4): 431–35.

60. Kamenícek, V., P. Holán, and P. Franěk. 2001. "[Systemic enzyme therapy in the treatment and prevention of post-traumatic and postoperative swelling]." *Acta chirurgiae orthopaedicae et traumatologiae Cechoslovaca* 68 (1): 45–49.

61. Secor, Eric R., Jr, Sonali J. Shah, Linda A. Guernsey, Craig M. Schramm, and Roger S. Thrall. 2012. "Bromelain Limits Airway Inflammation in an Ovalbumin-Induced Murine Model of Established Asthma." *Alternative Therapies in Health and Medicine* 18 (5): 9–17.

62. Brien, Sarah, George Lewith, Ann Walker, Stephen M. Hicks, and Dick Middleton. 2004. "Bromelain as a Treatment for Osteoarthritis: A Review of Clinical Studies." *Evidence-Based Complementary and Alternative Medicine: eCAM* 1 (3): 251–57.

63. Boss A, Bishop K, Marlow G, Barnett M, Ferguson L. Evidence to Support the Anti-Cancer Effect of Olive Leaf Extract and Future Directions. *Nutrients*. 2016;8(8). https://www.ncbi.nlm.nih.gov/pubmed/27548217.

64. Abunab H, Dator W, Hawamdeh S. Effect of olive leaf extract on glucose levels in diabetes-induced rats: A systematic review and meta-analysis. *J Diabetes*. 2017;9(10):947-957. https://www.ncbi.nlm.nih.gov/pubmed/27860303.

65. Lockyer S, Rowland I, Spencer J, Yaqoob P, Stonehouse W. Impact of phenolic-rich olive leaf extract on blood pressure, plasma lipids and inflammatory markers: a randomised controlled trial. *Eur J Nutr*. 2017;56(4):1421-1432. https://www.ncbi.nlm.nih.gov/pubmed/26951205.

66. Vogel P, Kasper M, Garavaglia J, Zani V, de S, Morelo D. Polyphenols benefits of olive leaf (Olea europaea L) to human health. *Nutr Hosp*. 2014;31(3):1427-1433. https://www.ncbi.nlm.nih.gov/pubmed/25726243.

67. Boss A, Kao C, Murray P, Marlow G, Barnett M, Ferguson L. Human Intervention Study to Assess the Effects of Supplementation with Olive Leaf Extract on Peripheral Blood Mononuclear Cell Gene Expression. *Int J Mol Sci*. 2016;17(12). https://www.ncbi.nlm.nih.gov/pubmed/27918443.

68. Romero C, Medina E, Mateo M, Brenes M. Quantification of bioactive compounds in Picual and Arbequina olive leaves and fruit. *J Sci Food Agric*. 2017;97(6):1725-1732. https://www.ncbi.nlm.nih.gov/pubmed/27447942.

69. Booz G. Cannabidiol as an emergent therapeutic strategy for lessening the impact of inflammation on oxidative stress.

Free Radic Biol Med. 2011;51(5):1054-1061. [PubMed]

70. Rajesh M, Mukhopadhyay P, Bátkai S, et al. Cannabidiol attenuates cardiac dysfunction, oxidative stress, fibrosis, and inflammatory and cell death signaling pathways in diabetic cardiomyopathy. *J Am Coll Cardiol.* 2010;56(25):2115-2125. [PubMed]
71. Weiss L, Zeira M, Reich S, et al. Cannabidiol lowers incidence of diabetes in non-obese diabetic mice. *Autoimmunity.* 2006;39(2):143-151. [PubMed]
72. Izzo A, Borrelli F, Capasso R, Di M, Mechoulam R. Non-psychotropic plant cannabinoids: new therapeutic opportunities from an ancient herb. *Trends Pharmacol Sci.* 2009;30(10):515-527. [PubMed]
73. Shi P, Diez-Freire C, Jun J, et al. Brain microglial cytokines in neurogenic hypertension. *Hypertension.* 2010;56(2):297-303. [PubMed]
74. Zuardi A. Cannabidiol: from an inactive cannabinoid to a drug with wide spectrum of action. *Rev Bras Psiquiatr.* 2008;30(3):271-280. [PubMed]
75. Pertwee R. The diverse CB1 and CB2 receptor pharmacology of three plant cannabinoids: delta9-tetrahydrocannabinol, cannabidiol and delta9-tetrahydrocannabivarin. *Br J Pharmacol.* 2008;153(2):199-215. [PubMed]
76. Toth C, Jedrzejewski N, Ellis C, Frey W. Cannabinoid-mediated modulation of neuropathic pain and microglial accumulation in a model of murine type I diabetic peripheral neuropathic pain. *Mol Pain.* 2010;6:16. [PubMed]
77. Kim D, You B, Jo E, Han S, Simon M, Lee S. NADPH

oxidase 2-derived reactive oxygen species in spinal cord microglia contribute to peripheral nerve injury-induced neuropathic pain. *Proc Natl Acad Sci U S A.* 2010;107(33):14851-14856. [PubMed]

78. Malfait A, Gallily R, Sumariwalla P, et al. The nonpsychoactive cannabis constituent cannabidiol is an oral anti-arthritic therapeutic in murine collagen-induced arthritis. *Proc Natl Acad Sci U S A.* 2000;97(17):9561-9566. [PubMed]

79. Toth C, Jedrzejewski N, Ellis C, Frey W. Cannabinoid-mediated modulation of neuropathic pain and microglial accumulation in a model of murine type I diabetic peripheral neuropathic pain. *Mol Pain.* 2010;6:16. [PubMed]

80. Weiss L, Zeira M, Reich S, et al. Cannabidiol arrests onset of autoimmune diabetes in NOD mice. *Neuropharmacology.* 2008;54(1):244-249. [PubMed]

81. Pacher P, Beckman J, Liaudet L. Nitric oxide and peroxynitrite in health and disease. *Physiol Rev.* 2007;87(1):315-424. [PubMed]

82. Rajesh M, Mukhopadhyay P, Bátkai S, et al. Cannabidiol attenuates high glucose-induced endothelial cell inflammatory response and barrier disruption. *Am J Physiol Heart Circ Physiol.* 2007;293(1):H610-9. [PubMed]

83. El-Remessy A, Al-Shabrawey M, Khalifa Y, Tsai N, Caldwell R, Liou G. Neuroprotective and blood-retinal barrier-preserving effects of cannabidiol in experimental diabetes. *Am J Pathol.* 2006;168(1):235-244. [PubMed]

84. Maes M, Galecki P, Chang Y, Berk M. A review on the oxidative and nitrosative stress (O&NS) pathways

in major depression and their possible contribution to the (neuro)degenerative processes in that illness. *Prog Neuropsychopharmacol Biol Psychiatry*. 2011;35(3):676-692. [PubMed]

85. Song C, Wang H. Cytokines mediated inflammation and decreased neurogenesis in animal models of depression. *Prog Neuropsychopharmacol Biol Psychiatry*. 2011;35(3):760-768. [PubMed]

86. El-Alfy A, Ivey K, Robinson K, et al. Antidepressant-like effect of delta9-tetrahydrocannabinol and other cannabinoids isolated from Cannabis sativa L. *Pharmacol Biochem Behav*. 2010;95(4):434-442. [PubMed]

87. Zanelati T, Biojone C, Moreira F, Guimarães F, Joca S. Antidepressant-like effects of cannabidiol in mice: possible involvement of 5-HT1A receptors. *Br J Pharmacol*. 2010;159(1):122-128. [PubMed]

88. Brown, Greg, John J. Albers, Lloyd D. Fisher, Susan M. Schaefer, Jiin-Tarng Lin, Cheryl Kaplan, Xue-Qiao Zhao, Brad D. Bisson, Virginia F. Fitzpatrick, and Harold T. Dodge. 1990. "Regression of Coronary Artery Disease as a Result of Intensive Lipid-Lowering Therapy in Men with High Levels of Apolipoprotein B." *The New England Journal of Medicine* 323 (19): 1289-98.

89. Martin, David L. 1994. "Pyridoxal Phosphate, GABA and Seizure Susceptibility." In *Biochemistry of Vitamin B6 and PQQ*, 343-47. Birkhäuser Basel.

90. Miodownik, Chanoch, Vladimir Lerner, Tali Vishne, Ben-Ami Sela, and Joseph Levine. 2007. "High-Dose Vitamin B6 Decreases Homocysteine Serum Levels in Patients with

Schizophrenia and Schizoaffective Disorders: A Preliminary Study." *Clinical Neuropharmacology* 30 (1): 13–17.

91. Cattaneo, Marco. 2017. "Hyperhomocysteinemia, Atherosclerosis and Thrombosis." *Thrombosis and Haemostasis* 81 (02): 165–76.

92. Nelen, W. L., H. J. Blom, E. A. Steegers, M. den Heijer, C. M. Thomas, and T. K. Eskes. 2000. "Homocysteine and Folate Levels as Risk Factors for Recurrent Early Pregnancy Loss." *Obstetrics and Gynecology* 95 (4): 519–24.

93. Put, N. M. van der, H. W. van Straaten, F. J. Trijbels, and H. J. Blom. 2001. "Folate, Homocysteine and Neural Tube Defects: An Overview." *Experimental Biology and Medicine* 226 (4): 243–70.

94. Dietrich-Muszalska, Anna, Joanna Malinowska, Beata Olas, Rafal Głowacki, Edward Bald, Barbara Wachowicz, and Jolanta Rabe-Jabłońska. 2012. "The Oxidative Stress May Be Induced by the Elevated Homocysteine in Schizophrenic Patients." *Neurochemical Research* 37 (5): 1057–62.

95. Morris, Martha Savaria. 2003. "Homocysteine and Alzheimer's Disease." *Lancet Neurology* 2 (7): 425–28.

96. Smach, Mohamed Ali, Nelly Jacob, Jean-Louis Golmard, Bassem Charfeddine, Turkia Lammouchi, Leila Ben Othman, Hedi Dridi, Soufien Bennamou, and Khalifa Limem. 2011. "Folate and Homocysteine in the Cerebrospinal Fluid of Patients with Alzheimer's Disease or Dementia: A Case Control Study." *European Neurology* 65 (5): 270–78.

97. Walsh, William J. 2014. *Nutrient Power: Heal Your Biochemistry and Heal Your Brain*. Revised, Updated ed. edition. Skyhorse.

Chapter 9 - Serotonin

1. "Declassified." n.d. Accessed April 2, 2021. https://web.archive.org/web/20020131081305/http://www.michael-robinett.com/declass/c011.htm.
2. Mansnerus, Laura. 1996. "Timothy Leary, Pied Piper Of Psychedelic 60's, Dies at 75." *The New York Times*, June 1, 1996. https://www.nytimes.com/1996/06/01/us/timothy-leary-pied-piper-of-psychedelic-60-s-dies-at-75.html.
3. AlterNet. 2017. "He Was No Hippie: Remembering Manson, Prison, Scientology and Mind Control." Raw Story - Celebrating 16 Years of Independent Journalism. November 26, 2017. https://www.rawstory.com/2017/11/he-was-no-hippie-remembering-manson-prison-scientology-and-mind-control/.
4. Babenko, V., P. Svensson, T. Graven-Nielsen, A. M. Drewes, T. S. Jensen, and L. Arendt-Nielsen. 2000. "Duration and Distribution of Experimental Muscle Hyperalgesia in Humans Following Combined Infusions of Serotonin and Bradykinin." *Brain Research* 853 (2): 275–81.
5. Hamel, E. 2007. "Serotonin and Migraine: Biology and Clinical Implications." *Cephalalgia: An International Journal of Headache* 27 (11): 1293–1300.
6. "Can-Long-Term-Antidepressant-Use-Be-Depressogenic.pdf." n.d. https://www.madinamerica.com/wp-content/uploads/2011/11/Can-long-term-andtidepressant-use-be-depressogenic.pdf.
7. Goldberg, D., M. Privett, B. Ustun, G. Simon, and M. Linden. 1998. "The Effects of Detection and Treatment on the

Outcome of Major Depression in Primary Care: A Naturalistic Study in 15 Cities." *The British Journal of General Practice: The Journal of the Royal College of General Practitioners* 48 (437): 1840–44.

8. https://www.nejm.org/doi/full/10.1056/NEJMsa065779
9. Kirsch, Irving, Brett J. Deacon, Tania B. Huedo-Medina, Alan Scoboria, Thomas J. Moore, and Blair T. Johnson. 2008. "Initial Severity and Antidepressant Benefits: A Meta-Analysis of Data Submitted to the Food and Drug Administration." *PLoS Medicine* 5 (2): e45.
10. Moncrieff, J., S. Wessely, and R. Hardy. 2004. "Active Placebos versus Antidepressants for Depression." *Cochrane Database of Systematic Reviews*, no. 1: CD003012.
11. Moncrieff, J., S. Wessely, and R. Hardy. 1998. "Meta-Analysis of Trials Comparing Antidepressants with Active Placebos." *The British Journal of Psychiatry: The Journal of Mental Science* 172 (March): 227–31; discussion 232–34.
12. Khan, A., H. A. Warner, and W. A. Brown. 2000. "Symptom Reduction and Suicide Risk in Patients Treated with Placebo in Antidepressant Clinical Trials: An Analysis of the Food and Drug Administration Database." *Archives of General Psychiatry* 57 (4): 311–17.
13. Leon, A. C. 2000. "Placebo Protects Subjects from Nonresponse: A Paradox of Power." *Archives of General Psychiatry*.
14. Turner, Erick H., Annette M. Matthews, Eftihia Linardatos, Robert A. Tell, and Robert Rosenthal. 2008. "Selective Publication of Antidepressant Trials and Its Influence on Apparent Efficacy." *The New England Journal of*

Medicine 358 (3): 252–60.

15. Frick, Andreas, Fredrik Åhs, Jonas Engman, My Jonasson, Iman Alaie, Johannes Björkstrand, Örjan Frans, et al. 2015. "Serotonin Synthesis and Reuptake in Social Anxiety Disorder: A Positron Emission Tomography Study." *JAMA Psychiatry* 72 (8): 794–802.
16. Zuardi, A. W. 1990. "5-HT-Related Drugs and Human Experimental Anxiety." *Neuroscience and Biobehavioral Reviews* 14 (4): 507–10.
17. Zimmerman, D., H. E. Abboud, L. E. George, A. J. Edis, and T. P. Dousa. 1980. "Serotonin Stimulates Adenosine 3',5'-Monophosphate Accumulation in Parathyroid Adenoma." *The Journal of Clinical Endocrinology and Metabolism* 51 (6): 1274–78.
18. Santos, Lucinéia dos, Telma G. C. S. de Andrade, and Frederico G. Graeff. 2010. "Social Separation and Diazepam Withdrawal Increase Anxiety in the Elevated plus-Maze and Serotonin Turnover in the Median Raphe and Hippocampus." *Journal of Psychopharmacology* 24 (5): 725–31.
19. Boer, Sietse F. de, and Jaap M. Koolhaas. 2005. "5-HT1A and 5-HT1B Receptor Agonists and Aggression: A Pharmacological Challenge of the Serotonin Deficiency Hypothesis." *European Journal of Pharmacology* 526 (1–3): 125–39.
20. Perry, George, Marta A. Taddeo, Akihiko Nunomura, Xiongwei Zhu, Tania Zenteno-Savin, Kelly L. Drew, Shun Shimohama, Jesús Avila, Rudolph J. Castellani, and Mark A. Smith. 2002. "Comparative Biology and Pathology of Oxidative Stress in Alzheimer and Other Neurodegenerative

Diseases: Beyond Damage and Response." *Comparative Biochemistry and Physiology. Toxicology & Pharmacology: CBP* 133 (4): 507–13.

21. Medvedev, A. E. 1990. "[Regulation by biogenic amines of energy functions of mitochondria]." *Voprosy meditsinskoi khimii* 36 (5): 18–21.
22. Hiroi, Ryoko, Ross A. McDevitt, and John F. Neumaier. 2006. "Estrogen Selectively Increases Tryptophan Hydroxylase-2 mRNA Expression in Distinct Subregions of Rat Midbrain Raphe Nucleus: Association between Gene Expression and Anxiety Behavior in the Open Field." *Biological Psychiatry* 60 (3): 288–95.
23. Hansenne, M., and M. Ansseau. 1999. "Harm Avoidance and Serotonin." *Biological Psychology* 51 (1): 77–81.
24. Graeff, F. G., M. B. Viana, and P. O. Mora. 1997. "Dual Role of 5-HT in Defense and Anxiety." *Neuroscience and Biobehavioral Reviews* 21 (6): 791–99.
25. Anthony, M. 1984. "Serotonin Antagonists." *Australian and New Zealand Journal of Medicine* 14 (6): 888–95.
26. Aleksandrin, V. V., N. N. Tarasova, and I. A. Tarakanov. 2005. "Effect of Serotonin on Respiration, Cerebral Circulation, and Blood Pressure in Rats." *Bulletin of Experimental Biology and Medicine* 139 (1): 64–67.
27. Lacasse, Jeffrey R., and Jonathan Leo. 2005. "Serotonin and Depression: A Disconnect between the Advertisements and the Scientific Literature." *PLoS Medicine* 2 (12): e392.
28. https://www.nejm.org/doi/full/10.1056/NEJMsa065779
29. Yokogoshi, H., Y. Kato, Y. M. Sagesaka, T. Takihara-Matsuura, T. Kakuda, and N. Takeuchi. 1995. "Reduction

Effect of Theanine on Blood Pressure and Brain 5-Hydroxyindoles in Spontaneously Hypertensive Rats." *Bioscience, Biotechnology, and Biochemistry* 59 (4): 615–18.

30. Yokogoshi, H., M. Mochizuki, and K. Saitoh. 1998. "Theanine-Induced Reduction of Brain Serotonin Concentration in Rats." *Bioscience, Biotechnology, and Biochemistry* 62 (4): 816–17.

Chapter 10 - How To Eat Thermo

1. Center for Food Safety, and Applied Nutrition. n.d. "Health Claim Notification for Whole Grain Foods." Accessed April 2, 2021. https://www.fda.gov/food/food-labeling-nutrition/health-claim-notification-whole-grain-foods.
2. Lee, Cheng-Sheng. 2015. *Dietary Nutrients, Additives and Fish Health*. John Wiley & Sons.
3. Oatway, Lori, Thava Vasanthan, and James H. Helm. 2001. "PHYTIC ACID." *Food Reviews International* 17 (4): 419–31.
4. Volek, J. S., W. J. Kraemer, J. A. Bush, T. Incledon, and M. Boetes. 1997. "Testosterone and Cortisol in Relationship to Dietary Nutrients and Resistance Exercise." *Journal of Applied Physiology* 82 (1): 49–54.
5. Hämäläinen, E., H. Adlercreutz, P. Puska, and P. Pietinen. 1984. "Diet and Serum Sex Hormones in Healthy Men." *Journal of Steroid Biochemistry* 20 (1): 459–64.
6. Bélanger, A., A. Locong, C. Noel, L. Cusan, A. Dupont, J. Prévost, S. Caron, and J. Sévigny. 1989. "Influence of Diet on Plasma Steroids and Sex Hormone-Binding Globulin Levels in Adult Men." *Journal of Steroid Biochemistry* 32 (6): 829–33.

7. Mascioli, E. A., B. R. Bistrian, V. K. Babayan, and G. L. Blackburn. 1987. "Medium Chain Triglycerides and Structured Lipids as Unique Nonglucose Energy Sources in Hyperalimentation." *Lipids* 22 (6): 421–23.
8. "What Is Oxidative Stress?" 2010. March 2, 2010. https://www.news-medical.net/health/What-is-Oxidative-Stress.aspx.
9. Yoshikawa, Toshikazu, and Yuji Naito. 2002. "What Is Oxidative Stress?" 2002. https://www.med.or.jp/english/pdf/2002_07/271_276.pdf.
10. "Arsenic In Your Food Investigated - Consumer Reports." n.d. Accessed April 2, 2021. https://www.consumerreports.org/cro/magazine/2012/11/arsenic-in-your-food/index.htm.
11. Chris Kresser, M. S. 2012. "Arsenic in Rice: How Concerned Should You Be?" Chris Kresser LLC. October 12, 2012. https://chriskresser.com/arsenic-in-rice-how-concerned-should-you-be/.
12. Bressani, Ricardo, Juan Carlos Turcios, Ana Silvia Colmenares de Ruiz, and Patricia Palocios de Palomo. 2004. "Effect of Processing Conditions on Phytic Acid, Calcium, Iron, and Zinc Contents of Lime-Cooked Maize." *Journal of Agricultural and Food Chemistry* 52 (5): 1157–62.
13. Dombrink-Kurtzman, M. A., T. J. Dvorak, M. E. Barron, and L. W. Rooney. 2000. "Effect of Nixtamalization (Alkaline Cooking) on Fumonisin-Contaminated Corn for Production of Masa and Tortillas." *Journal of Agricultural and Food Chemistry* 48 (11): 5781–86.
14. "Interciencia - Revista Interciencia." n.d. Accessed April 2, 2021. https://www.interciencia.net/.

15. Pappa, María Renée, Patricia Palacios de Palomo, and Ricardo Bressani. 2010. "Effect of Lime and Wood Ash on the Nixtamalization of Maize and Tortilla Chemical and Nutritional Characteristics." *Plant Foods for Human Nutrition* 65 (2): 130–35.
16. https://naldc.nal.usda.gov/download/23799/PDF
17. https://www.aaccnet.org/publications/cc/backissues/1992/documents/69_275.pdf

Made in the USA
Columbia, SC
09 March 2023